Leadership for Person-Centred Dementia Care

Buz Loveday

Foreword by Professor Murna Downs

Jessica Kingsley *Publishers*
London and Philadelphia

Figure 1.2 on p.23 from Kitwood 'Person and Process in Dementia' has been reproduced with permission from the *International Journal of Geriatric Psychiatry*. Figure 1.6 on p.35 has been reproduced with permission from the Bradford Dementia Group. Figure 3.2 on p.71 from the Dementia Care Leadership Programme has been reproduced with permission from the Bradford Dementia Group. Figure 4.1 on p.89 from Kolb (1983) was adapted with permission from Peter Honey Publications.

First published in 2013
by Jessica Kingsley Publishers
116 Pentonville Road
London N1 9JB, UK
and
400 Market Street, Suite 400
Philadelphia, PA 19106, USA

www.jkp.com

Library of Congress Cataloging in Publication Data
A CIP catalog record for this book is available from the Library of Congress

British Library Cataloguing in Publication Data
A CIP catalogue record for this book is available from the British Library

ISBN 978 1 84905 229 0
eISBN 978 0 85700 691 2

Printed and bound in Great Britain

For Molly, Daniel and Mojo

In loving memory of my grandmother
Margaret Loveday,
known as 'Doidle'

Contents

Foreword by Professor Murna Downs   9

Acknowledgements   11

Introduction: Beginning the Journey   13

Chapter 1 Focusing on the Goals of Person-Centred Dementia Care   19

Chapter 2 Identifying the Barriers to Person-Centred Care   43

Chapter 3 Empowering and Supporting Staff   65

Chapter 4 Creating a Learning Culture: The Role of Training and Reflective Practice   83

Chapter 5 Ensuring Effective Communication with Staff, Families and Professionals   107

Chapter 6 Working Together to Respond to Feelings and Needs   127

Conclusion: Moving Forward   147

References   151

Index   155

Foreword

This book *Leadership for Person-Centred Dementia Care* could not come at a better time. We are in the midst of a political groundswell of support for transforming the quality of care for people with dementia and their family carers. There is now widespread recognition that to live well with dementia requires an informed and effective workforce – across all levels and sectors – guided and supported by effective leaders. For over 20 years Buz Loveday has provided training and workforce development to care teams to help them realise the potential of person-centred dementia care. In this book she shares with us this wealth of expertise and experience.

In *Leadership for Person-Centred Dementia Care* Buz takes us through the key elements of both person-centred dementia care and leadership skills. She takes a refreshing approach to leadership arguing that in learning organisations, managers are not the only leaders. Rather, leadership occurs, and is required, at all levels of the organisation. Indeed one of the roles of managers is to identify and nurture these natural leaders.

This book provides a timely and grounded overview of the key skills required of leaders and how these skills can be acquired and enhanced. I have no doubt that *Leadership for Person-Centred Dementia Care* will become one of the cornerstones guiding our movement to ensure that people live well with dementia.

Professor Murna Downs
Series Editor of Bradford Good Practice Guides Dementia Group
University of Bradford

Acknowledgements

Many have supported and encouraged me along the way, but I am especially grateful to two people in particular. First, Murna Downs, for her ongoing encouragement and unwavering belief in my ability to write this book, not to mention her patient advice and many constructive suggestions that shaped it into a cohesive whole. Second, Sue Heiser, who read the drafts and contributed much insightful wisdom borne from her extensive experience as a leader in dementia care.

Without the friendship, guidance and inspiration of the late Tom Kitwood I doubt this book would ever have come to be, but then I can't imagine the world of dementia care without Tom's work. It was certainly through him that my interest in dementia care leadership first developed – an interest that has continued to grow over the years, fuelled by the many dedicated and passionate leaders I've been lucky enough to meet and work with along the way, not to mention the even greater numbers of dedicated and passionate dementia care staff who struggle without effective leadership. I am indebted to Sue Harrison and David Parry for their strong commitment to developing the ability of care home managers to put their knowledge into practice and make person-centred dementia care a reality. It was they who first commissioned the development and delivery of my training course, the Dementia Care Leadership Programme, on which this book is largely based.

In writing this book I have drawn extensively on the experiences and insights shared by many managers and other leaders who have attended my training courses – particularly participants on the Dementia Care Leadership Programme, the Dementia Care Trainers' Programme and the Dementia Champions leadership development programme. So many of their ideas and stories fill the pages of this book – I'm hugely appreciative and sorry not to be able to mention them all by name. I would just like to give one specific mention to Helen Browne, who gave me the little gem of 'www.ebi'.

My thanks go also to my training associates and friends Brenda Bowe, Janet Lallysmith and Jo Savill – their unstinting drive and determination to improve dementia care is vital not only in making Dementia Trainers successful but also to me on a personal level for brainstorming, debriefing, problem-solving and generally charging my batteries. On which note, all my friends and family deserve my heartfelt gratitude for helping me have fun, offload and stay connected with the rest of my life during the process of writing this book, with a special thank you to my very good friend Carol Frankl for also telling me about the Learning Walk.

Introduction
Beginning the Journey

It is estimated that by 2030 there will be 65.7 million people with dementia worldwide (Alzheimer's Disease International 2009). It is a priority to focus on how we can best provide care. Over recent years, dementia care has been going through a slow but steady process of transformation – a huge body of evidence now exists about ways of enabling people with dementia to live well, and increasingly we encounter examples of excellent and innovative practice. But the transformation is by no means complete. Many dementia care services have not changed in any significant way for decades, and others are trying but struggling.

It was in 1995 that Tom Kitwood first wrote of a 'new culture of dementia care' and the creation of this new culture is still very much a work in progress – one that is huge, daunting and also potentially exhilarating. It is not a journey that can be undertaken single-handedly; nor is it one that is likely to be completed quickly. But with effective leadership it is possible for any dementia care service to embark on the road towards excellence.

In order to lead a staff team towards best practice in dementia care, it is essential to have a vision – a clearly formed idea of where the care service is heading and how it will look once it has arrived. Equally, it is vital to understand that there will always be work to do to maintain the positive momentum. Even when goals have all been achieved, there is more to do: there will always be new challenges to meet, new ideas that emerge. Leading a dementia care service takes energy and determination. It requires a passionately held belief that every person with dementia can be supported to live well, with senses of self-worth and identity; feelings of security and acceptance. It also requires a deep understanding that it is only through nurturing, guiding and supporting the staff team that the needs of people with dementia can be met. Passion on its own is not enough. A leader also needs the skills to make it happen.

THE AIM OF THIS BOOK

This book aims to highlight the key features of dementia care leadership, focusing on *what leaders need to know* and *what leaders can do* to develop person-centred dementia care services. It is a practical book rather than a theoretical one, with lots of examples to bring the ideas to life. I hope that whatever kind of dementia care leadership role you have, you will find within it things that you can make use of to help you think through your own leadership approach – what you could do more of, what you could do differently and what new techniques you could implement to develop and improve person-centred dementia care.

Much of this book reflects the content of training courses I have developed and delivered for leaders over recent years – particularly the accredited Dementia Care Leadership Programme. I have focused on what participants on these courses have found to be relevant and useful, and many of the examples I give are drawn from their work, helping to show how ideas can be implemented in real-life situations.

The leaders I've worked with on these courses have had a variety of job roles ranging from service managers to care staff. This book is aimed at the same wide range of leaders.

It is not just for managers, although it will certainly be relevant to them, but other staff within care services can also play key roles in dementia care leadership and this book is for them too. Dementia care services need more than one leader. Indeed, I hope that you are not the only person from your care service who will be reading this book or considering the issues it covers, because developing a person-centred culture of care is too big an undertaking for one leader to achieve single-handedly.

The kind of leadership that can be offered from people working within the care team is an invaluable supplement to the dementia care leadership provided by managers. Such roles are often known as 'Dementia Champions' – motivated staff members who have been nominated to take on particular responsibilities for influencing dementia care. Such individuals are in a prime position to role model excellence in their interactions with and care of people with dementia and they can mentor less experienced staff, offer informal advice and encouragement, and help their fellow team members develop their understanding of individuals. Dementia Champions are likely to be highly aware of the realities of the team's work and the challenges currently faced; their advice and guidance will always be grounded in reality.

CONTENT

For some readers of this book, many of the ideas will be very familiar. I have pulled together some key themes of person-centred care and considered them from a leader's perspective. I have drawn on the work of those who have inspired me – people such as Tom Kitwood, Christine Bryden and Graham Stokes – added some ideas drawn from spheres of social psychology, management and education, mixed them together with wisdom drawn from the practical experiences of many inspired and dedicated dementia care leaders I have met along the way, and finally dropped in a few thoughts of my own.

In Chapter 1, I explore some of the key goals for dementia care. If you're leading people, you must know where you're taking them, so it is particularly important that you have a clear concept of what you are aiming to achieve for the people with dementia receiving care from your service. I consider the leader's role in relation to each of these goals and introduce some ideas about the type of leadership approach most likely to bring them to fruition.

In Chapter 2, I look at some obstructions to person-centred care, such as negative attitudes, unhelpful norms and outdated policies. I focus on some of the ways in which dementia care leaders can work to identify and combat these barriers.

In Chapter 3, I examine various aspects of the leader's role in empowering and supporting staff, beginning with the importance of role modelling. I consider how you can get the best from staff, and the importance and practicalities of providing emotional support. The chapter concludes by looking at ways of promoting effective teamwork.

In Chapter 4, I focus on the importance of ongoing learning for person-centred dementia care, getting the best value from any training that is provided and helping staff learn from their experiences with people with dementia. I explain some effective techniques that you can use to facilitate reflective practice.

In Chapter 5, I look at the various verbal and written communication processes that are necessary for person-centred practice, and what leaders can do to maximise the effectiveness of these. I then consider how to create positive working relationships with other professionals and how to support and involve families and friends of people with dementia.

In Chapter 6, I consider some types of situations that challenge dementia care staff and how leaders can support the development of enhanced practice. I consider some particular challenges for leaders that arise when risk is involved and look at practical ways of upholding people's best interests.

I conclude by facing forward, thinking about the first steps that can be taken towards the achievement of your vision. It might be a long road ahead but what's important is that you're heading in the right direction. I very much hope that this book will serve as a useful guide.

Chapter 1

Focusing on the Goals of Person-Centred Dementia Care

By the end of this chapter, you will:

- Recognise some key goals of dementia care:
  - minimising secondary losses of ability
  - maximising potential
  - maintaining personhood
  - addressing the needs of the whole person
  - optimising well-being.
- Have considered the leader's approach and their role in relation to these goals.
- Understand the importance of communicating a vision and making this apparent in day-to-day priorities.

'A leader is a dealer in hope.'

Napoleon Bonaparte (cited in Holden 1988)

If a care service is person-centred, this means that it values each and every person involved with it – everyone matters. People with dementia are right at the core, and the care that is provided is effectively determined by them. The focus is not on theories about 'what works' or 'what's good for people with dementia', but is on the individual men and women receiving care and support and what they – as individuals – need and want.

Thus person-centred care is freeform in shape; there's no guidebook that can accurately tell staff what to do, because the only way of discovering what to do is through learning about each individual. There are no short-cuts – staff require energy, resourcefulness and commitment, and they must have a clear concept of where they are heading. They need to understand that it is completely possible for people with dementia to have a high quality of life, and they must recognise their own power and influence over this.

RECOGNISING GOALS FOR DEMENTIA CARE

Through the work of Tom Kitwood (1997), Dawn Brooker (2007) and others, the last decade of the twentieth century and the first decade of the twenty-first saw a revolution in our understanding of dementia. It is now widely accepted that dementia does not have to be the hopeless diagnosis that it once was. Indeed, the National Dementia Strategy for England is titled *Living Well with Dementia* (Department of Health 2009). Even though there is still no cure, there is much that can be done to enhance well-being and enable people with dementia to maximise their potential.

Minimising secondary losses of ability

While it is important to understand at least a little about how the brain is affected by the diseases that cause dementia, it is invariably a mistake to assume that all the difficulties experienced by an individual with dementia are symptoms of this neurological impairment alone. To make this assumption is to fall prey to 'diagnostic overshadowing' – the assumption that all of a person's difficulties can be attributed to their diagnosed condition. Just as a person with a mobility problem can be made more disabled by the physical and social environment that surrounds them, the difficulties experienced by people with dementia often have multiple causes (see Figure 1.1).

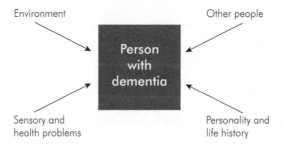

Environment

Other people

Person with dementia

Sensory and health problems

Personality and life history

Figure 1.1: Possible causes of difficulties experienced in dementia

External factors, particularly when combined with the real symptoms of dementia, can contribute many additional problems – or 'secondary losses of ability' (Jolley 2005, p.27).

For example

A new environment is likely to increase the disorientation of an individual who is already experiencing some memory problems.

Dim lighting is likely to contribute to perceptual difficulties.

A noisy environment can inhibit communication.

Disempowering care practice (for example doing something for a person that they would have been able to do themselves) can cause an individual to start to lose their own abilities through lack of use.

The disorientation, perceptual difficulties, communication problems and loss of abilities mentioned in these examples are not symptoms of dementia, but secondary losses of ability. Recognising this is vitally important because it opens up the possibility of improvement. Such losses of ability can be reversed and, with sufficient awareness, they can even be prevented from occurring in the first place.

We must also consider the individual's own personality and life history and how these may influence their experience of dementia.

For example

A very private person, who has lived alone all her life, may well find the experience of having to accept help with personal care to be extremely distressing – this could then lead to agitated behaviour or withdrawal.

Equally it is important not to overlook the effects of health problems, sensory deficits and physical disabilities on cognitive functioning.

For example

The experience of being in pain can easily cause a shorter attention span, restlessness or confusion, and is one of the key reasons for verbal or physical aggression.

So to enable people with dementia to function as well as possible, there needs to be an ongoing focus on identifying and eliminating the causes of secondary losses of ability. The role of the dementia care leader is to reflect and question; to refuse to accept that the person's dementia is inevitably the reason for every difficulty that they experience. You should approach such problems with a belief that there are probably other causes to be found, and that these can be tackled, enabling a person's functioning to improve.

Kitwood (1993) illustrated the gap between a person's actual functioning and the maximum possible level of functioning given the structural intactness of the brain (see Figure 1.2).

He explained that the challenge for good dementia care is to enable a person's functioning to improve towards the upper limit. Eradicating factors causing secondary losses of ability would effectively mean closing this gap (see Figure 1.3). This outcome is one of the key goals in the care of people with dementia.

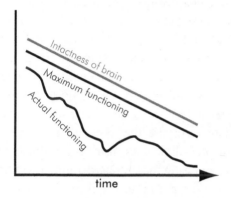

Figure 1.2: Course of a dementing illness (Kitwood 1993)

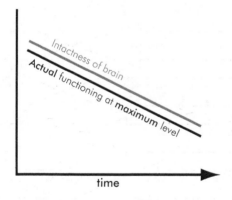

Figure 1.3: Optimal course of a dementing illness

Maximising potential

While we can aim to close the gap between maximum and actual functioning, unfortunately there is nothing that can be done to arrest the continuing decline in the intactness of the brain. But even though we cannot eliminate symptoms caused by this decline, there is much that staff can do to help the person function despite them. If staff work to compensate for the person's difficulties, through taking on parts of a task that the person can no longer do, they can help to alleviate or avoid the frustration, embarrassment and damage to self-esteem that the person would experience each time they 'failed' to do it themselves. And while doing the parts of a task that the person with dementia cannot do, staff must enable the person to fully use their remaining abilities, thus undertaking every task jointly with the person with dementia – working in partnership – so that the person can feel a sense of achievement (see Figure 1.4). It is essential to recognise that every person with dementia, however severe their difficulties, also has abilities and strengths. It is through recognising these strengths and providing multiple opportunities for the person to use them that staff can enable the person to feel good about themselves and their life.

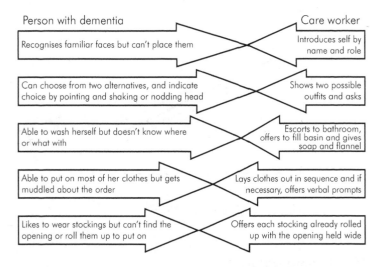

Person with dementia — Care worker

Recognises familiar faces but can't place them — Introduces self by name and role

Can choose from two alternatives, and indicate choice by pointing and shaking or nodding head — Shows two possible outfits and asks

Able to wash herself but doesn't know where or what with — Escorts to bathroom, offers to fill basin and gives soap and flannel

Able to put on most of her clothes but gets muddled about the order — Lays clothes out in sequence and if necessary, offers verbal prompts

Likes to wear stockings but can't find the opening or roll them up to put on — Offers each stocking already rolled up with the opening held wide

Figure 1.4: Maximising potential through working in partnership

Here a key role of the dementia care leader is to ensure that effective systems are in place for the ongoing assessment of people's strengths and needs. The processes of assessment and care planning are explored in Chapter 5. Clearly, though, it is not enough simply to have information on file about what a person can and cannot do – you must make explicit the expectation that all support given to each individual will be based on that person's abilities and difficulties. All staff must be made aware that their role is not to 'do for' but to 'do with', and the way they care for each person will inevitably be different to the way they care for other people, for no two individuals will have exactly the same abilities, difficulties and preferences.

Maintaining personhood

Of the many myths that form barriers to good dementia care, one of the most insidious is the assumption (to be considered further in Chapter 2) that dementia robs people of their identity and personality. This is far from true. In fact it is only through a detailed understanding of who a person is and the life they have been leading that they can be truly understood and their needs met.

Thus the gathering of detailed information about the individual is key – their cultural and social background, their values and beliefs, their preferences and interests. Not only does this information enable staff to act in accordance with the person's individual needs, but also it enables them to value each person as an individual and see things from their perspective, understand their feelings and take them very seriously. The information can also be used as a starting point for life story work, an activity that can be highly valuable in helping to affirm and boost the person's own sense of their personhood. A life story could take a variety of different guises, from a scrapbook to a box of memorabilia, and can be something that is gradually created with the person with dementia over a period of weeks or even months. Useful guidance can be found in Murphy (1994).

Dementia care leaders must prioritise the process of information gathering from the first point of contact with the individual, finding out as much as possible from the person themselves, families, friends, members of the individual's community and other professionals. Crucially, the process must involve front-line staff, who, through building trusting relationships with those they are supporting, will have multiple opportunities to encourage the person to share information about themselves. Staff who are supporting people living in their own homes can often learn much about their client as an individual from noticing and perhaps starting conversations about things in the person's environment, such as photos and ornaments.

Staff must be encouraged to pay very close attention to everything the person with dementia communicates verbally, non-verbally and through their actions – for example, their responses to choices offered will often provide valuable information about their preferences. There may be times when the only information available is what can be discovered from the person with dementia themselves.

For example

Debbie Christian (1997) wrote a moving account of her work with Ruby, who had arrived at the nursing home as little more than a list of challenging behaviours and with no background information. Christian described how, through lowering her own barriers, she entered into Ruby's subjective reality, engaged with her with openness and tenderness, and found the humorous, purposeful and loving individual that lay behind the misunderstood behaviours.

So the dementia care leader needs to be the champion of the person who lies behind the symptoms and behaviours, ensuring that all possible steps are taken to discover and connect with the unique individual who is invariably still there.

Once the person is known, every interaction can be personalised – and can therefore help to maintain the individual's sense of personhood – from helping the person carry out their religious rituals, to ensuring that the right brand of hand soap is placed on their wash basin. The person's environment, too, should help to maintain personhood. When people live at home, their environment is likely to support their sense of identity, as long as the person remains in charge of their own space. There is a risk that when a person becomes a 'service user' and their home becomes someone's workplace, changes are made by professionals and carers and the individual starts to lose their sense of control. In care homes and day centres it is particularly important for the environment to be tailored to the people living or spending time there. Furnishings and decor should represent the cultural backgrounds, interests and eras that are most familiar to clients. Individuals' rooms in care homes should be highly personalised – it is the person's bedroom, more than any other space within the care setting, that is their 'home'. People should have control over their own personal space – such as having a key to the door of their own room – and the freedom to move around the building and find where they want to go. There should be no unnecessary restrictions, like toilets marked 'staff only', and when restrictions are genuinely necessary because of safety risks, it is much better to reduce the visibility of such areas – for example by painting the door the same colour as the wall (Pool 2007) – rather than making people aware that they are being excluded. Further ways in which the environment can help to minimise risk are covered in Chapter 6.

Addressing the needs of the whole person

The bodily needs of people with dementia must be given full attention. From the importance of identifying medical concerns, to the care that must be taken to properly address people's day-to-day physical needs like nutrition and hygiene, dementia care services have essential responsibilities in relation to people's physical well-being.

Psychological well-being is also vital. Fundamental to the development of a person-centred dementia care service is the priority that must be given to addressing the psychological needs of people with dementia for comfort, attachment, inclusion, identity and occupation (Kitwood 1997). These needs are addressed primarily through the way staff communicate and the relationships they develop.

Person-centred care is a relationship-based approach. Being a person-centred carer involves being a person first and a professional second, relating to the person with dementia as one human being to another. All human beings need to feel accepted, understood and important and this is all the more urgent because of the emotional vulnerability dementia causes. Thus it is vital that staff both help people to maintain the relationships that they have with family and friends, and also provide this much-needed closeness themselves, since many people with dementia spend considerably more time with their professional carers than with anyone else in their lives. So person-centred caring involves developing connections, demonstrating not only respect, but also love. As David Sheard (2007) says, person-centred is not something you 'do', but rather is something you 'are'.

Such relationships need to be genuine – to come from the heart. This means that staff have to draw on their own personal resources and involve their own emotions, which ultimately makes care work much more fulfilling but it can also be personally draining and challenging, potentially confronting staff with their own vulnerabilities and difficult feelings. Staff members will not be able to provide and maintain such relationships unless they are able to express their feelings to someone who listens and understands what it's like for them. So dementia care leaders need to be prepared to appreciate and empathise with staff, and work to develop relationships with them to enable them to connect deeply with people with dementia. This aspect of leadership will be considered further in Chapter 3.

The poet Maya Angelou said that although people are likely to forget what you said and did, they always remember how you make them feel. These words teach a vital lesson to all those involved in dementia care: staff have a profound and lasting influence on the feelings of people with dementia. Christine Bryden, writing from the first-hand perspective of someone living with dementia, stresses the importance of this when she tells us: 'It's the way you talk to us, not what you say, that we will remember. We know the feeling, but don't know the plot' (Bryden 2005, p.138).

Thus every moment of contact that staff have with a person with dementia is significant and can have a positive or negative effect. Staff need to communicate at every possible opportunity, from a brief greeting as somebody passes by, to a lengthy conversation while

In your care service:

Are clear explanations given to people with dementia to enable them to make choices and fully understand what's going on?

Do staff chat with warmth and humour, prepared to share information about their own lives if this would be of interest to the person they're talking to?

Is every care task used as an opportunity for communication?

Do staff search for ways of making contact with individuals who are withdrawn?

Are feelings always attended to, however they may be communicated?

Are staff able to recognise expressions of need that hide behind apparently 'delusional' utterances, such as the need for safety and security that may be expressed through crying out for 'mother'?

someone is being helped to eat a meal. And they need to understand that the content of this interaction quite possibly matters less than the key message that they should convey through every interaction they have: that the person matters to them. Leaders need to emphasise

> Do staff take seriously the messages communicated through a person's behaviour, working to understand and respond to these just as they would to any other form of communication?

that positive communication is a priority and be keenly aware of the kinds of communication that are actually taking place.

It is also important that staff should help people with dementia to engage with the world around them. For the vast majority of people without dementia, everyday life is filled with busy-ness, from mundane chores, to satisfying leisure pursuits, to work, but in contrast, the lives of many people with dementia are empty and unfulfilling. In any situation where a person with dementia is receiving care, there are many small and larger opportunities to support them to be engaged and occupied. You need to ensure that all staff understand the importance of this for people with dementia, and help them think of ways in which they can use their time with people to address this need. Even though time is limited, any contact that staff have with people with dementia – even personal care – can be a stimulating experience for the client if staff approach it with the right attitude. It is very important that occupation is seen as the responsibility of all staff who are involved with people with dementia – not just as the role of one single staff member, professional group or care setting.

For example

The home care worker who offers the service user a tea-towel to dry the dishes while she washes up.

The handyman who asks a resident to help him fix a dripping tap.

The care worker who helps a resident to choose one of her CDs to listen to as she is assisted to get ready for bed each evening.

What is important is to build on the person's abilities and interests, to provide an antidote to the low self-esteem and other difficult feelings often experienced by people with dementia. However many abilities a person has lost, there are always some things that they are still able to do, and doing something together with a staff member or other clients provides an excellent context for the development of relationships.

The physical surroundings can also help to address psychological needs. Sheard (2008, p.57) has written about how the environment can support the need for occupation, for example, by having lounges 'full to the brim with everyday items which can be touched, held, fiddled with or passed around, smelt or tasted'. It is important that lighting, seating arrangements and noise levels enable people to easily communicate with each other and that group environments offer variety, with different places where people can chat, relax, be alone, be with others, be occupied, watch TV or have a view of the world outside. Having ready access to outside space is important for many people, and the way garden areas are designed can enable people to derive maximum pleasure and stimulation from being there (Chalfont 2008).

Optimising well-being

When Baroness Warnock stated her belief that huge numbers of people with dementia would 'much prefer to die rather than continue in the state they are in' (BBC News 2008) and suggested that they are 'wasting people's lives' because of the care they require (Beckford 2008), she failed to understand something that is fundamental: even though higher mental functioning declines in dementia, the point of existence is not simply to achieve – the value of a human being and the quality of their life goes far beyond their cognitive ability.

A key determinant of quality of life is not so much what you can do, but how you feel. If we think about some of the times in our life when we have had the most positive feelings, we will find that many are unrelated to our cognitive abilities. For example the feelings of warmth and security that come from knowing that we are loved or the sense of self-worth we experience when we are listened to and respected. The vast majority of people living with dementia are also capable of having these feelings, as long as the support they receive meets their psychological as well as their physical needs. Thus the closer staff come to fully meeting a person's needs, the higher the level of well-being they are likely to engender. Bearing witness to this can be hugely encouraging and motivating for staff, so it is of high importance that staff know what signs to look for and understand the strong correlation between well-being and their positive input.

We have already considered that two key objectives in the care of people with dementia are to facilitate the highest possible level of functioning and to uphold personhood. Leading on from these is the ultimate aim for dementia care leaders – that of maintaining people's well-being even as dementia progresses (Kitwood and Bredin 1992a). This is illustrated in Figure 1.5 alongside the goal of maximising functioning described earlier in this chapter.

One way that we can recognise that a person with dementia is experiencing a sense of well-being is by observing how they engage with the world – people are likely to be alert and act with evident purpose; they will often show some concern about other people, perhaps through attempting to be helpful. We can look for signs of confidence, which we might recognise when we see a person using their remaining abilities, initiating verbal or non-verbal interactions with other people or expressing themselves creatively, for example through music or dance. We can also notice well-being through the person demonstrating their self-respect, maybe through showing concern for their own privacy, or taking pride in their achievements or appearance. A person experiencing well-being will feel a sense of control over their own life, and we will know this because they find a way of making their presence felt, and do what they can to express their wishes and needs. This person will not necessarily cooperate with what we want them to do, but rather will insist that we cooperate with them. Integral to well-being will be the person's relationships with others: the person finds a way of connecting with other people, expresses affection, shows humour, and experiences trust, contentment and relaxation.

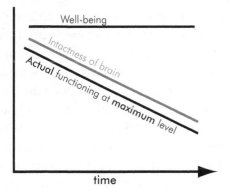

Figure 1.5: Maintaining well-being

For example

Betty receives home care support to help her get ready each morning, but if the agency ever sends a carer that Betty doesn't know well, she refuses assistance and turns them away. Once she gets to the day centre, Betty tends to make herself busy, helping to push the tea trolley and collecting the empty cups when people have finished. She chats with other clients, and sometimes makes jokes. Betty can often be seen adjusting her clothing or combing her hair.

Well-being does not mean that the person is in a state of continuous happiness, but they will certainly not be unremittingly depressed, anxious or angry. If this is the case, we need to be concerned – the person is in a state of ill-being and it is likely that this has come about because they have unmet psychological or physical needs. Dementia care leaders hold responsibility for the well-being of the people with dementia receiving care from their service. You must be keenly aware of how each individual is faring, through quickly recognising signs of met and unmet needs. When individuals are showing signs of ill-being you must battle against any assumptions that this is part of an inevitable decline and be determined to find ways of enhancing the person's well-being.

Of course, leaders will not be able to achieve this single-handedly. You need to ensure that staff are aware of the different ways in which people with dementia might indicate their ill-being and well-being, and are encouraged to look for these signs. Witnessing signs of ill-being, and being aware that these are not symptoms of dementia, can help to foster a determination within the team to identify and address the person's unmet needs. Seeing evidence of well-being provides essential feedback and validation for their work. There will be far greater motivation to work well when the results of doing this are apparent.

Moreover, looking for signs of well-being and signs of ill-being helps staff to see the communication and behaviour of people with dementia in a different light. What might once have been considered as a problem – for example, the individual who assertively refuses to accept personal care from the new home carer who she hasn't met before – can now be seen as something positive, in that the individual is clearly expressing her wishes and demonstrating her self-respect. It is up to the home care service to find a way of providing care in accordance with the person's wishes and needs.

Using, on a regular basis, a tool such as the Bradford Well-being Profile (Bradford Dementia Group 2008), part of which is reproduced in Figure 1.6, can be very useful in helping staff pay attention to signs that might otherwise have been missed, and gradual trends that could have gone unnoticed.

BRADFORD WELL-BEING PROFILE: POSITIVE INDICATORS

(To be used in conjunction with the guidelines in the Bradford Well-being Profile)

Name:	Observers:		Date:

Positive indicators	Strong	Weak
1 Can communicate wants, needs and choices		
2 Makes contact with other people		
3 Shows warmth or affection		
4 Shows pleasure or enjoyment in daily life		
5 Alertness, responsiveness		
6 Uses remaining abilities		
7 Creative expression (e.g. singing, dancing)		
8 Is co-operative or helpful		
9 Responds appropriately to people/situations		
10 Expresses appropriate emotions		
11 Relaxed posture or body language		
12 Sense of humour		
13 Sense of purpose		
14 Signs of self-respect		

Figure 1.6: Bradford Well-Being Profile: Positive indicators
Source: reproduced with kind permission from Bradford Dementia Group (University of Bradford 2008)

INSPIRING AND GUIDING STAFF

There is so much potential for people with dementia to live well despite their disability, and responsibility for making this happen lies with dementia care leaders. Leadership is not simply about managing a team; indeed, dementia care leaders may not even hold management positions. Rather, leadership is about holding a vision, and inspiring and guiding movement towards it.

In order to inspire, you need to be trusted and respected by your team. Thus person-centred leadership is not about exerting authority but is about being congruent, involved and 'walking the walk' as well as 'talking the talk'. In *Dementia Reconsidered* (1997), Kitwood wrote that an organisation that is committed to the personhood of people with dementia must also be committed to the personhood of its staff. This means that leaders must listen and respond to the experiences and feelings of individual staff members, and do so with empathy rather than judgement. Person-centred leaders do not set themselves up on a pedestal of superiority and infallibility but they work to enable staff to create their own strategies, find their own answers and develop their own skills and insights. They value staff for who each person is and what they bring to their work, and they understand what each staff member may need from them. These aspects of dementia care leadership will be explored throughout the subsequent chapters of this book.

Creating a shared vision

It is commonplace nowadays for organisations to have vision or mission statements – the difference between the two being that while a mission statement focuses on an organisation's objectives, a vision focuses on its aspirations. But too often, such statements are no more than a series of catchphrases. The term 'person-centred', for example, has been used so often, and to mean so many different things, that it is in danger of losing its meaning altogether. The Kings Fund principles of choice, dignity, respect, independence and privacy (1986) have long been embedded in the language used to talk about dementia care, but, sadly, are frequently contradicted in practice.

In order for a vision to be more than just words, it needs to be based on specific goals, which you passionately believe can be achieved. One of the many challenges for person-centred dementia care leaders is that too often their hopes and ambitions are not shared by enough people and a 'yes but...' mentality prevails, where the barriers to the achievement of these goals are seen as insurmountable. But the stronger and more distinct your vision of the future and the more heartfelt your communication of it, the more inspired your staff team will be to work towards achieving it. If you can create a vivid and compelling image, and articulate this so that everyone else can see and feel it, this creates drive and energy – you help staff see how every single aspect of their day-to-day work;

> **Visualisation**
>
> This is the future – imagine that you are visiting the care setting where you currently work...the positive momentum that has started from the changes you are making now has continued, and everything that you could dream of in relation to the lives of your clients has been achieved... it is truly a wonderful place to be...the well-being of both clients and staff is at an all-time high...people with dementia could not be leading a better life...imagine that you walk in the front door and look around you... What do you see people with dementia doing? What do you see staff doing? ...be in that place, looking around you... What's happening?... What do you feel?... Now begin to walk around the building... What do you see?... What do you hear?...

every task they undertake, is ultimately in service of this vision. Effective teamwork is grounded in such shared goals, where individuals fully understand their personal responsibilities and roles in bringing them to life.

The greater the part that individuals play in creating a vision, the more likely this is to happen. A powerful activity to carry out with your team is a visualisation exercise (see visualisation panel for example) whereby individuals dare to dream of a utopian future for their care service – the products of such unleashed imaginations can provide powerful antidotes to complacency and pessimism.

Making priorities clear

When a vision is shared, everyone is pulling in the same direction and there is also a common understanding of day-to-day priorities. For example, all staff in the care home will appreciate that attending to a resident's emotional needs is more important than making beds; that a successful mealtime is one where residents have socialised, engaged and taken their time, rather than one that has been completed as quickly as possible.

It is for the leaders of person-centred dementia care to make priorities explicit, ensuring that there is consistency in the expectations verbally communicated by all senior staff and that these are also evident in the organisation's written policies and procedures. If an organisation's vision genuinely informs the day-to-day activities that take place within it, every written document must reflect this. The health and safety procedure must include measures that can be taken to support freedom of movement and reasonable risk-taking. Individuals' care plans must be holistic, and focus on the person's strengths and abilities as well as their difficulties and disabilities. And if an organisation is serious about promoting well-being, there must be clear guidelines on action that can be taken to protect the rights of service users, from a watertight whistleblowing system, to a clear and effective disciplinary procedure.

The recruitment procedure is of particular importance when it comes to making priorities clear. Job descriptions should make explicit that communication with people with dementia is a central feature of every job role within the care service; person specifications must document the qualities and abilities needed to be person-centred. Patience, empathy, respect and enthusiasm, for example, are essential qualities and should, therefore, be listed as 'essential criteria'. It is important to think about how to draw out these qualities during the recruitment process. Where possible, it is helpful to involve people with dementia in the process of recruitment. This could involve introducing prospective recruits to service users with dementia, perhaps as part of a tour around the care home or day centre conducted by an experienced staff member who is able to assess the person's attitudes. If there is someone who is able to do so, it can be highly beneficial to involve a person with dementia on an interview panel.

> Consider the person specification for dementia care staff within your organisation – does it reflect the skills and qualities necessary for person-centred care? Do job descriptions include how the post holder will be expected to address the psychological needs of people with dementia?

The wording of job advertisements and the questions that are asked at an interview can be very important in finding the right people. 'Can you dance?' was a question posed to potential job applicants at one care home, for example. It was not that the ability to dance would, in itself, determine whether or not the applicant was recruited, but their answer to the question would certainly demonstrate something about their attitudes. 'No, but I can sing!' might suggest an individual who is prepared to give something of themselves to their work, whereas 'But I thought this was an interview for a care work job' would indicate something very different about what the person was able and willing to bring to the role.

Many organisations require job applicants to have prior experience in care work, but you should consider whether this is really a necessary – or even desirable – criterion. People may well have developed bad habits in previous jobs and, as I will consider in Chapter 2, 'unlearning' bad information and changing habits is a much more arduous process than learning good knowledge and approaches in the first place. Increasingly, organisations serious about person-centred care are recognising that recruiting staff with no prior experience in dementia care might be the best way of ensuring that they are recruiting staff who are free of bad habits.

MAKING IT POSSIBLE

Not only must priorities be made explicit, but also they must be made possible, through allocating sufficient time and resources. However, as I will explore in Chapter 2, there are numerous barriers to person-centred care and shortage of resources is generally top of the list. Making real a person-centred philosophy within a limited budget and with insufficient time involves skilful and creative management.

For example

One care home manager recognised how some residents were being rushed at mealtimes because the level of needs was high and there was an insufficient number of staff. No money was available in her budget to increase staffing numbers, but the effective solution she found was to split mealtimes into two sittings.

In another care home, changing the time of the main meal of the day to the evening rather than lunchtime resolved the problem that many residents, having spent their afternoon asleep after a heavy lunch, had been restless and sometimes agitated in the evenings, when staff were busy helping other people to bed and had no time to provide occupation.

Flexible thinking is important in ensuring that person-centred practice is prioritised – sometimes it is by noticing and changing an unhelpful procedure or routine that staff time can be freed up to address people's needs more effectively. In so many care homes, for instance, morning personal care is rushed because of an unnecessarily rigid breakfast time. Lengthening the time during which breakfast is available can relieve the stress for both residents and staff. And sometimes in home care service provision, even though the length of a visit cannot be extended, it may be that something achievable like changing the time of the visit could enable improved practice.

For example

A home care coordinator shifted one client's morning visit from 9 a.m. to 8 a.m. This meant that rather than battling with the client to remove the clothes she had already put on without washing, the carer arrived when the client was still in her nightclothes and could prompt her towards the bathroom.

Thus in their efforts to inspire and support a team to pull together towards the achievement of their vision, dementia care leaders must remain focused on day-to-day practicalities and individual situations. It will not be possible to change a culture of care overnight, and by its very definition a vision is something distant that determines the direction of travel. On the journey there, dementia care leaders need to think creatively about how to enable people to give their best and ensure that existing resources are used to maximum benefit.

Table 1.1 Chapter 1 key points

Key points	What leaders need to do
Person-centred care is highly flexible and guided by goals	Keep talking about these goals, helping staff relate their input to the bigger picture
The difficulties experienced by people with dementia can be caused by a range of factors	Lead staff in searching for and addressing the causes of people's difficulties
Through working in partnership with people with dementia, staff can help to maximise potential	Ensure that clients' abilities and needs are known and that staff know their role is to 'do with'
It is a priority to help people with dementia maintain their personhood	Enable staff to learn about individuals and personalise their care and the environment
Meeting psychological needs must be seen as a priority	Support staff to develop positive relationships and help them find the best ways of using their time with individuals
The ultimate goal in dementia care is to enhance well-being	Recognise evidence of well-being and ill-being, help staff to recognise this too and use it to validate good work and identify needs
Person-centred care requires person-centred leadership	Reflect on your leadership approach and ensure that it demonstrates what you want to see staff doing
Leaders should clearly define a vision for the future of their care service	Create and describe a vivid and compelling image of how it will be when the goals are achieved
The vision must guide day-to-day priorities and procedures	Make priorities explicit – for example when recruiting staff – and ensure they can be implemented

Chapter 2

Identifying the Barriers to Person-Centred Care

By the end of this chapter, you will:

- Recognise barriers to person-centred care and be able to identify your role as a leader in tackling them:
  - negative attitudes
  - group norms
  - individual habits
  - hopelessness
  - unhelpful policies, procedures and systems
  - limited resources.
- Understand how observation and discussion can help to prompt awareness of what needs to change.

Person-centred leadership requires an open heart and an open mind; a commitment to honest and open reflection; a willingness to listen to feedback from all sources and recognise and admit where there are problems. Perfection doesn't exist in the real world and a leader who feels that there's no room for improvement within her or his care service has become complacent and grown oblivious to aspects of the care service that could be better.

RECOGNISING BARRIERS

There are multiple barriers to person-centred care, and a central function of dementia care leadership is to identify and dismantle them. This is no easy task. The barriers range from deep-seated beliefs of individuals to institutionalised ageism made manifest in systems and procedures, and are apparent in many aspects of dementia care. Kitwood described 17 types of damaging care practice, which he termed 'malignant social psychology' (Kitwood 1997) and which include infantilisation, mockery and outpacing. While rarely carried out with the deliberate intention of causing harm, these practices, sadly still rife in dementia care environments, undermine the well-being and diminish the personhood and abilities of people with dementia. Understanding the reasons for such poor practices, and the nature of the obstacles that can block the route to person-centred care, is the first step to tackling them.

Negative attitudes

Let us first consider those who work in the front line – the individual staff members who are in day-to-day contact with people with dementia – and the attitude with which they approach their work and their clients. Attitudes are influenced by a range of factors including knowledge and beliefs. A lack of understanding about the symptoms of dementia, for example, can lead to the mistaken belief that a person is being deliberately difficult, and an ensuing impatient attitude that results in dismissive or even abusive behaviour. Since the progressive brain damage occurring in dementia is not evident from the outside, people's symptoms and needs can be easily misunderstood in a way that would be unlikely to happen if the damage was more visible. Some knowledge about the way the brain changes in dementia is, therefore, important in appreciating a person's difficulties and developing an empathic attitude.

But knowledge about neurological impairment and its resulting symptoms is by no means all that's needed. In fact, another area of information is far more important: knowledge about the individual men and women with dementia who are receiving care.

For example

If we are to care for Mahmud, we need to understand who he is. How has he lived his life? What has been important to him? What and who have been the key events, people, occupations, achievements, routines and habits that have shaped how he has lived his life? What can we understand about his personality, emotions, culture, religion, sexuality, views, interests, preferences, superstitions, phobias and relationships?

Person-centred care can take place only if staff are committed to the ongoing process of gathering and using this knowledge in Mahmud's care (the importance of ongoing assessment and strengths-based care planning are fully explored in Chapter 5). But more than this: the apparently simple act of finding out about someone's life can have quite a profound effect on the attitudes of care staff, enabling them to see beyond the dementia to recognise, understand and fully appreciate the person who is living with the condition.

It is worth noting that in order to learn about dementia, many people first need to 'unlearn'. Even those who believe they know much about dementia are likely to have been exposed to a host of misinformation and negativity. Much of what we hear and read about dementia in the media suggests that those living with the condition lose their identity, worth and any possibility of leading a good quality life. Dementia is described, for example, as something that robs people of their identities (Social Care Institute for Excellence (SCIE) 2009), or as 'the death that leaves the body behind' (Kitwood 1997, p.3). Such negative views of dementia are pervasive and damaging, influencing opinions and creating a sense of hopelessness that will have an unfortunate effect on the care approach. After all, what's the use of getting to know Miriam if she has lost her identity? How could Donald have any emotional needs if everything other than his body has already died?

Unfortunately it's not only journalists who perpetuate destructive views on dementia. It is also still common to hear negative opinions from doctors and other medical professionals. Since there is no medical cure for a primary dementia such as Alzheimer's disease, a pessimistic prognosis is understandable, but too often this is presented in a way which denies the possibility of living well with dementia. Doctors' opinions are generally held in high regard and as such are very influential. So the medical verdict that 'there's nothing that can be done for her' can easily contribute to subliminal beliefs of care staff and subsequently have quite a profound impact on the social care approach.

> What words and phrases about dementia have you encountered in the media? How might these influence people's attitudes towards those living with dementia?

Staff levels of motivation are also likely to be affected by general views on the condition their clients experience. After all, if you believe you are caring for those for whom 'nothing can be done', you are likely to feel that your work is mundane and unimportant. Many staff identify themselves as 'just a care worker'. With such low morale, they will have little incentive to put in any extra effort or be creative. Dementia care leaders need to be sensitive to the feelings experienced by staff who are involved in the care of people with dementia, because the way they feel about their clients, their colleagues and their role will shape their attitudes and approach. This area is explored further in Chapter 3.

Ajzen and Fishbein (2005, p.206) explained that 'Implicit attitudes – being automatically activated – ...guide behaviour by default unless they are overridden by controlled processes'. It is vital, then, for dementia care leaders to implement 'controlled processes', such as training and coaching (to be considered in Chapter 4), to ensure that staff are supported to shed any implicit negative views and recognise how much potential there is to enhance the quality of life of their clients – how much, therefore, they can achieve in their work.

Group norms

Since the early 1990s, a host of inspirational writing and research has promoted an alternative, positive picture of what is possible in dementia care. Care for people with dementia is now widely recognised as an exciting, innovative and fruitful area of work. Many of those entering the field of dementia care more recently will be starting out with a positive outlook. But in many care homes and other dementia care services, long-entrenched norms – or group habits – exist, grounded in a lack of respect, a set of negative assumptions and institutionalised routines. Task-centred, rather than person-centred, approaches are still common where priority is given to the delivery of personal care and domestic chores, while psychological needs are often unnoticed or disregarded. Perhaps it is not surprising that such unhelpful approaches persist. As recently as the 1960s this was the widely accepted norm for dementia care (Adams 2008) and

> The Alzheimer's Society *Home from Home* report in 2007 found that the average amount of time that people with dementia in care homes spent interacting with staff or other residents (excluding care tasks) was two minutes in every six hours. How do you think this compares to the norm in your own care service?

it was not until the 1990s that a new culture of person-centred care was promoted by pioneers such as Kitwood (1997) and Kitwood and Benson (1995). There are many staff in post, of all grades, who have worked within dementia care services in the same or a similar job for many years, and when a care worker has previously been told off for talking to residents 'when there are beds that need to be made', they are likely to have internalised a powerful message about priorities.

Dementia care leaders need to be aware of the power of group norms and conformity. You may have heard new staff being told 'This is how we do it here'. This can result in the positive attitudes and good intentions demonstrated at interview being diverted to a different course of action. Newly recruited staff can lack the confidence to go against the group norm as they do not wish to be excluded from the group or face conflict. The famous Asch experiment in the early 1950s demonstrated the human tendency to conform to group norms (Asch 1951). We have all experienced situations in which we have felt reluctant to single ourselves out by going against a trend – being the only hungry wedding guest to tuck in to the lavish buffet before the allocated time, for example!

It is a potentially uncomfortable situation for staff who are aware that the care approach they are adopting is different from the one they have intended to implement. Faced with this kind of incongruity, the human mind will try to minimise the 'cognitive dissonance' that arises and, since it would be too challenging to break with the norm, the person adjusts their attitude to fit with their new behaviour (Festinger 1957). Thus the new staff member, only weeks ago so full of promise, becomes indistinguishable from the rest of the team in both their approach and their attitudes.

The nature of norms is such that all too often they are not thought about. Staff just act in a certain way because 'we've always done it that way' and the lack of conscious consideration is followed by a lack of conscious reflection, so the same mistakes occur again and again, the same negative outcomes arise, and no-one stops to wonder why.

For example

All residents have showers at Steely House Care Home, and these showers take place before breakfast, which is served at 8.30 a.m. Some of the residents are 'aggressive' before or during their shower, which means that staff have to work in pairs. The experience for staff is at best dispiriting and at worst injurious; the experience for residents is distressing, depersonalising and abusive. But that's the way it's done at Steely House, so no-one has investigated residents' hygiene preferences or wondered why some people are aggressive; there is no suggestion that people's hygiene needs could sometimes be met at other times of the day, or – shock horror! – that people who wanted to could get up later!

In some group care settings it is still the unquestioned norm that the TV is on all day while people with dementia sit slumped around the edge of the room, withdrawn and unresponsive. Should anyone stand up they are told to sit down. They all wear pads and are 'toileted' at fixed times. In one care setting I encountered (a long-stay hospital ward), the patients were all deprived of their false teeth and ate pureed food, because there was a perceived risk of choking (more on the assessment and management of risk in Chapter 6).

Group norms are powerful in their capacity to influence behaviour, and yet they rarely stand up to much scrutiny. Even just drawing people's attention to them can prove to be a powerful strategy. The dementia care leader can simply ask the staff team why, for example, they consider it to be so important that all residents should be washed and dressed by 8.30 a.m. and what would be the worst that could happen if this were not achieved.

In order to overcome group norms, dementia care leaders need to consider ways of replacing their rewards. For example, one of the rewards for staff practising a task-centred approach to care is the satisfaction of seeing the visible results of the tasks they have completed – the clean and nicely dressed resident, for example, or the neatly made bed. The results of person-centred care are far more important, but less evident. For example, it perhaps takes more attuned awareness to notice the previously anxious individual who now feels much more relaxed as a result of her keyworker listening to and comforting her. Dementia care leaders can increase the rewards of person-centred work merely by noticing and commenting on the results. 'Myrtle is so much more relaxed since you spoke with her earlier', for example. Ensuring that staff are familiar with observable evidence of well-being (see Chapter 1) will also help to validate positive care practice. The importance of validating positive work is explored further in Chapter 4.

It is important to consider the most effective way of making changes. Patience is an important virtue. Leaders who try to transform their service too rapidly risk overwhelming the staff team and leaving people feeling no sense of control over what is going on. Just as we can outpace people with dementia we can outpace our staff teams, which will prevent staff from being able to embrace new ideologies or methods. Fossey and James (2008) found that too much change at once decreases motivation for change, as does a culture where staff are fearful of making mistakes. Leaders must give careful thought to how they can bring the team with them through the process. Evidence analysed by Fossey and James (2008) indicated that key motivational factors for change are an awareness of what's currently wrong and a readiness to learn and develop, thus leaders must foster these conditions as an essential component of the process of change management.

Individual habits

Our behaviour is influenced not only by what those around us are doing, but also by what we are used to doing ourselves – our own habits. A habit is a behavioural pattern that is learnt through being repeated regularly. It is a very basic form of learning that usually occurs without conscious thought. Forming a habit tends to be much easier than changing one – the latter process tends to require a concerted, highly conscious effort. Individual staff habits play an important part in determining the quality of care practice. Helping staff to develop positive person-centred care habits is an important function of dementia care leaders.

Some poor care is the result of individual habits that have been left to develop unchecked. Not bothering to ask whether people would like tea or coffee, for instance; failing to knock when entering a resident's room; speaking to colleagues over the heads of people with dementia. Since habits are

> When is the last time you gave up a habit? How did you manage it? Did you use any strategies that could be applied to the endeavour of helping staff give up bad habits?

hard to break, leaders will need to exercise patience and offer frequent reminders when trying to encourage staff to change such habits. It is helpful if these reminders are free from blame, because if the staff member feels blamed they will probably become defensive and then their motivation will be to avoid getting into trouble again (being more careful when they're being watched), rather than to have any personal commitment to changing their bad habit. The more staff are encouraged, without feeling censured, to be consciously aware of what they are doing; the more often they are prompted to think about why they are doing it that way and how their approach might impact on those they are caring for, the more likely they are to let go of negative behavioural patterns.

Habits also inhibit creative thinking. Staff get stuck in a rut – they keep on doing the same thing simply because that's the thing they're used to doing. The more often a habit is practised, the deeper the rut becomes, the steeper the sides, and the harder it is to keep sight of alternative courses of action. Thus the Vera Lynn CD is always played after breakfast in the first floor lounge. Two of the residents seem to like it, five ignore it and/or fall asleep, three show signs of distress and one person usually leaves the room to walk up and down the corridor. Maybe when the CD was first played (15 years ago) Vera Lynn had a larger fan-base in the first floor lounge (or maybe no-one thought about it then either). But one thing that's pretty certain is that in another 15 years' time there will be even fewer Vera Lynn aficionados, so someone had better dig the way out of that rut soon!

Hopelessness

The 'stuck in a rut' process easily happens at a management level too.

For example

One care home manager complained that the relatives of most of her residents were unwilling to share information about the person's background and life story. The manager felt that she was doing all she possibly could – relatives were given a form to fill in before the new resident moved in. If they didn't fill in the form, a staff member would attempt to go through the questions with them on the phone, or face-to-face once the resident moved in. Most relatives left sections of the form blank, provided only sparse information for the sections they did fill in, and refused to share much more information verbally. The manager had reached a point of hopelessness, having drawn the conclusion that relatives were simply unwilling to divulge information.

Taking an overview, it seems quite apparent that if the strategy of asking relatives to fill in the form wasn't working, there were a number of things to rethink and alternative courses of action that could be tried. It could have been the way the form was worded, for example – were the questions sufficient to guide relatives as to what information would be helpful? It could have been the way the form was introduced to them – perhaps there was insufficient explanation as to why the information was needed and how it would be used. Maybe using a form simply wasn't the best method of gathering the breadth and depth of information required. Or perhaps it was a matter of timing – asking for detailed information before the relative has grown to trust the care home is actually requiring a big leap of faith. Moreover, requiring this information at exactly the time when the relative is likely to be in the throes of deep emotions (just before or just after their loved one has moved into a care home) is unlikely to harvest the best results.

Climbing out of the rut involves suspending hopelessness and considering the possibility that solutions can be found. This takes significant effort and enough resilience to ride through setbacks and treat them as learning opportunities. The more specific we can be about precisely what it was that did and didn't work, the more we are equipped to decide whether any of the strategies already used are worth trying again. Perhaps, for example, the relatives' form did tend to bring useful results from relatives who had lived with the person with dementia for some time before they moved into the care home? Perhaps there was one question on the form that was usually answered well?

It is almost always useful to start small when trying to bring about a change. Keep the long-range goals in mind, but focus your attention on the multiple small steps that will need to be taken en route. Concentrating on these will bring many benefits – not least that the process becomes manageable and there are many opportunities for small achievements that can boost morale and increase motivation.

For example

Let's start with Liz – the wife of Bernard, a new resident – and focus on one area of information that she has not addressed fully on the form; let's say this is the section about interests and hobbies.

1. The manager begins by chatting to Bernard's keyworker and encouraging her to think about some of the ways that residents' lives are enhanced through using information about their hobbies and interests.

2. The manager asks the keyworker to share some of these examples with Liz.

3. The manager phones Liz to ask if she would be so kind as to spend a little time with the keyworker on her next visit.

4. The manager allocates some time for the keyworker to spend with Liz to chat about Bernard's interests.

If the keyworker succeeds in gathering any further information from Liz about Bernard's interests and hobbies then she's achieved something really important. The manager, too, can feel more confident now that solutions to the problem do exist, and the small success can fuel her determination to carry on finding them. If the planned approach with Liz has been unsuccessful, the manager and keyworker can sit down together to think about it, learn from it, and plan what to try next.

Thus new habits can be developed – those involving cooperative problem-solving and reflective practice. This will be explored further in Chapter 4.

Unhelpful policies, procedures and systems

We have earlier considered the group norms or culture that can exist within a staff team and how influential these can be in guiding care practice. Even more powerful are the norms that exist on an organisational level, guiding service provision and resource allocation. Let us take, as an example, group care settings that offer no flexibility over mealtimes – in such situations clients will inevitably be rushed, disempowered and denied choice. A primary contributor to the human rights abuses taking place on a daily basis at 'Steely House Care Home' (the example given earlier) was the fixed breakfast time. Added into the equation, quite possibly, were job descriptions that focused on tasks and a staffing rota that placed the responsibility for getting residents up and attending to their hygiene needs firmly on the morning shift of staff.

In some large unit-based care homes, I have come across a policy whereby all staff rotate around units on a regular basis, thereby destroying the possibility of residents growing to trust and feel safe with care staff they know. And I have encountered organisations where some of the operational procedures are quite obviously based on misinterpretations of legislation on important matters such as the protection of vulnerable adults, health and safety and data protection.

For example

A large care home provider that forbade staff from touching residents other than to give personal care – any other touch was considered 'abusive'.

A care home that deemed it unsafe for residents to be in the (enclosed) garden because they were perceived to be 'at risk of eating earth or stones'.

A home care agency where care staff were told nothing about new clients they went to visit – not even whether or not the person had dementia – because of 'confidentiality'.

Clearly such misguided policies lead to the needs of people with dementia being neglected.

An unhelpful management style can also pose barriers to person-centred care. When leaders exert high levels of power over their team members and staff are given few opportunities for making suggestions, a climate of resentment and apathy tends to grow. Staff are disempowered and feel that what they do or say does not really make a difference – thus less effort will be made, challenges will be avoided and potential creativity is wasted. Empowerment and mutual cooperation are fundamental to person-centred care and leaders who can draw on the experience and ideas of their team members will stand a far greater chance of making it happen.

Dementia care leaders who hold senior management positions need to be prepared to take risks, to challenge the status quo and use their influence within the organisation to make or advocate for changes to policies, procedures, systems and documentation. Depending on their role within the organisation, many leaders may be more limited in their ability to tackle organisational norms and routines, but it's essential to keep plugging away. Being a leader means sticking your neck out; lobbying for improvements even if you have no direct control over making them happen. Even if you are not a manager, you will have some knowledge about how things are currently done within your organisation, and who makes decisions. Speaking to the right person at the right time, ensuring that the views and needs of both people with dementia and the staff who are for them are heard, might well be the way of setting changes in motion. Be prepared to give descriptive examples of how things actually are and make suggestions about what could be done differently. If you present the case with enough knowledge and enough passion you will be heard.

Limited resources

While there are always things within the care setting that can be changed for the better, from improvements in individuals' attitudes to the rewriting of outdated policies, there are nearly always some factors contributing to poor care practices that lie outside of the leader's control. Top of the list would be resources – or the lack thereof. Funding limitations are potentially the biggest barrier of all to achieving the goals of person-centred dementia care. The reality is that rates of pay do not reflect the high level of skill necessary for person-centred dementia care, and staffing ratios are insufficient to give individuals the attention they need. It is a huge challenge for dementia care leaders to bring out the best practice possible given these restrictions. Sometimes even the basic physical needs of people with dementia are unavoidably neglected – if two people need help to go to the toilet at exactly the same time, for example, and one of the two care staff on shift is already helping somebody to have a bath. For home care services, a key determinant in guiding the care approach is the length of time allocated for each visit. Commonly, home care staff have visits of half an hour to assist the service user out of bed, help them go to the toilet, wash, dress and eat their breakfast. How is it possible, in this situation, for staff to avoid a task-focused approach to care?

I think the answer lies in how existing resources are used: given that they are currently insufficient, it is vital to work creatively to make the most of everything that is available even as we campaign for increases. Home care staff may always have too many tasks to achieve in too short a time, but how the tasks are undertaken will make a big difference for the person with dementia.

For example

The home care worker who fills the half hour with communication, empathy and humour, and enables the service user to do some small parts of her own personal care, demonstrates that a person-centred approach is still possible in limited situations.

This is not to say that outcomes are uncompromised – indeed, were more time available there would probably be more of her own personal care that the person with dementia could be supported to do

> Can you identify any ways in which staff could better use their time?

for herself and far more meaningful conversations that could develop. Leaders need to seize every opportunity to advocate for the needs of service users and make commissioners aware of any ways in which people are being disabled for want of extra time. But dementia care leaders also need to help staff find the most beneficial ways of using their limited time and empower them to be as creative and flexible as possible, in order to best respond to the service user's needs at any given moment.

In terms of the most important 'resource' of all – the staff working in dementia care – although only very few are paid in accordance with the true value and complexity of their work, still the profession manages to attract some truly outstanding carers. This is particularly so in organisations that maximise other motivational factors (more on this in Chapter 3). Creating a perfect team is likely always to be a work in progress, but it is not an impossible ambition for care services that nurture their staff with high levels of support and validation and invest in them with the very best in training and other developmental opportunities.

TAKING STOCK

As I wrote at the beginning of the chapter, dementia care leaders working towards person-centred care must be prepared to reflect honestly on the state of play within their care service. The first step towards change is to raise awareness of what it is that needs changing. Evidence of this can be found through observation, conversation with key stakeholders including people with dementia, staff and families, and audits of policies, procedures and care records.

While the process of gathering information can be delegated, it can be helpful for leaders to carry out observations and engage in conversations themselves. This can be done informally but it may be helpful to use structured methods for investigation. One such structured approach is Dementia Care Mapping (DCM) (Brooker and Surr 2005), a practice development methodology recommended by National Institute for Health and Clinical Excellence (NICE)/SCIE (2007). Developed specifically for embedding person-centred dementia care practice it involves briefing service users, families and staff, observing the experience of care from the perspective of the person with dementia, engaging staff teams in reflecting on the observations and joint action planning. The effectiveness of these plans is then assessed by starting the cycle again after a period of time.

Using a highly detailed and comprehensive observation measure of quality of life, DCM provides information about how people with dementia spend their time, their mood and engagement and the number and type of interactions with care staff which address psychological needs and maximise or undermine personhood. The National Audit Office (2010) recommended DCM as a useful observational measure of quality of life for people with dementia, and the approach has been widely used in health and social care settings nationally and internationally since the mid-1990s, to support the embedding of person-centred care in practice (Brooker *et al.* 1998; Martin and Younger 2001; Williams and Rees 1997). There is good evidence of its use in practice settings as a quality audit and improvement tool (Ballard and Aarsland 2009; Chenoweth *et al.* 2009).

While DCM provides highly detailed observational evidence, a general overview of care practices can be gained from a method such as the 'Learning Walk'. This technique is adapted from a model used within education services and created by the National College for School Leadership (2006). Candidates on my course, the Dementia Care Leadership Programme, used Learning Walks to form the structure of exchange visits which they undertook with a colleague (or a small group of colleagues) from another dementia care setting. A Learning Walk is basically a brief action research project. Its intention is not to evaluate and develop the quality of care in the way that DCM does, but simply to prompt professional reflection and learning. Undertaking this process in a pair or small group creates an opportunity to learn from different perspectives and thereby gather evidence that will help the leader of the dementia care service to identify evidence of progress and areas in need of development. Each leader also benefits from having a chance to observe and learn in a colleague's care setting, realising how things can be similar yet very different and seeing with fresh eyes aspects of the care setting that its own leader may not have recently noticed.

For example

One pair of leaders undertaking a Learning Walk noticed that for the whole time they spent in the care home lounge, two staff members were sitting in the room writing their daily notes and did not speak to residents once. Some residents spoke to each other once or twice, but there were many signs of boredom. In contrast, when the leaders sat in the dining room at lunchtime, there was much evidence of positive communication, from friendly banter to sensitive and discreet verbal prompts. Clearly staff knew how to communicate positively but did not understand that communication should take priority over paperwork, and had not been helped to find a more suitable time to write their notes without neglecting residents.

A Learning Walk is most useful if it focuses on a specific aspect of the care service. Dementia Care Leadership Programme candidates have used this method to investigate communication, relationships and engagement – key areas through which the attitudes of staff and the norms of the care approach are made manifest. The aim is to enable the dementia care leaders who undertake it to better understand the nature of communication and engagement within their care setting and the factors that positively contribute to it, and thereby develop a plan of action for enhancing it.

Before undertaking the observations it is important to agree on 'look-fors' that will provide evidence of positive communication, relationships and engagement. Being clear about what will be observed helps participants to get the most out of the project. Each Learning Walk involves short observations in different areas of the care setting, with reflective discussions taking place immediately after each observation, and also brief information gathering sessions with staff and visitors (if any are present). After a final debriefing session between the walkers during which developmental needs are discussed, an action plan is created, defining specific targets for enhancing communication, relationships and engagement within the care setting and the steps that can be taken to achieve them. A Learning Walk is a valuable opportunity to gain a deeper level of insight into the barriers to person-centred care and how to tackle these.

> What are some of the things you could look at that would provide evidence of positive communication between staff and people with dementia?
>
> What could you look for that might help you assess the quality of relationships between staff and people with dementia?

While observational methods such as the Learning Walk are helpful in group care settings, if your care service provides support for service users in their own homes, your opportunities to witness care practice are far more limited. In terms of direct observations, you will need to rely on prearranged situations such as shadowing, observations and reviews, which might not give a true impression of the everyday communication that takes place, although they still highlight the style of interactions and flag up the staff member's abilities for and understanding of good practice. One-to-one discussions with staff will often reveal much about the nature of the interactions that take place behind closed doors. Sometimes a true flavour of the worker's approach emerges through analysing a problem they have shared, with questions such as 'How did you explain what you were doing?' and 'What did you say to Mrs Rajan when she refused to get up?'.

CONCLUSION

There are many influences on dementia care practice and not all of them are within the control of the leader. However, what's important is to focus on making manageable changes and to celebrate achievements, however small. I am reminded of the sentiment of the 'Serenity Prayer', attributed to the theologian Reinhold Niebuhr (1987), which emphasises the need for serenity to be able to accept things we cannot change, for courage to make changes that are possible and for sufficient wisdom to be able to distinguish one from the other.

This could serve as a useful mantra for any dementia care leader.

Table 2.1 Chapter 2 key points

Key points	What leaders need to do
Poor attitudes stem from a lack of knowledge about dementia and individuals	Provide ongoing opportunities for learning and unlearning
In many dementia care services, there are task-focused norms that inhibit good practice	Initiate reflection by asking 'why'; replace pay-offs of task-focused care by validating person-centred practice; be patient
Staff can easily get into bad habits	Give frequent, blame-free reminders to prompt conscious awareness
Managers can get stuck in a rut and feel hopeless	Set realistic goals and concentrate on a step-by-step process of change
The policies, procedures and systems of the organisation can be blocks to person-centred care	Recognise such barriers when they exist and make or advocate for the necessary changes
Some factors that inhibit person-centred practice are outside of the leader's control	Make best use of existing resources and celebrate achievements
Leaders need a keen awareness of day-to-day practices in order to identify barriers to good care	Initiate qualitative audits and evaluations, observations and discussions

Chapter 3

Empowering and Supporting Staff

By the end of this chapter, you will:

- Recognise that it is essential for you to role model good practice.
- Understand how to empower staff to use their strengths and do their best.
- Recognise some important factors that motivate staff in dementia care.
- Understand the importance of drawing out and supporting leadership potential from within the staff team.
- Understand why and how to give emotional support to staff.
- Have thought through some strategies for building a cooperative team.

MODELLING PERSON-CENTRED CARE

As I mentioned earlier in this book, being a person-centred leader is about 'walking the walk' as well as 'talking the talk'. For a vision to be effectively communicated, it must guide everything you do and be apparent in everything you do. Leaders need to take seriously their responsibility as role models.

For example

The nursing home team leader who is seen always to take the time to chat to residents.

The day centre manager who is frequently witnessed letting go of her inhibitions and fully engaging in activities with clients.

Both of these leaders are setting powerful examples about expectations and feasibility. They demonstrate what is possible even when time is limited and resources are short, they model the nature of good communication and they reinforce the point that this is what all staff should be doing.

It is helpful for leaders to recognise that if you are trusted and respected by the staff team, potentially everything you do may be copied. Thus consistency and congruence are essential qualities of effective role models – clients' feelings are not suddenly disparaged when a visitor is present; the leader does not demonstrate respect when talking

> What are some of the things that staff have seen you doing over the last week? Would it be positive if they were to copy the attitudes and practices you have demonstrated? What might be lacking from their approach if they only did what they have seen you doing?

to people with dementia but then laugh about them behind their backs. The person-centred dementia care leader is unfailingly respectful towards people with dementia and everything that they do is guided by their attention to people's feelings and needs.

As role models, dementia care leaders need to spend as much time with people with dementia as possible. This is undoubtedly a challenge when there are many demands on your time, but while paperwork has to be completed, meetings attended and phone calls made, it is also vitally important that you are involved, on a regular basis, in the hands-on delivery of care. You must have very good knowledge of each client as an individual, particularly the person's background and their psychological needs. Leaders also need to have up-to-date awareness of what's happening with each service user, but you are not expected to know everything – rather, an important aspect of the leader's role modelling is that you are prepared to ask, to listen and to observe. It is right and proper that care staff, for example, will know more about the day-to-day details of an individual's life than will their manager; what is important is that the manager is inquisitive, interested and thoughtful, and thereby demonstrates the importance of questioning and reflection (more on this in Chapter 4). This also conveys something very important about empowerment – the leader who defers to a care worker for their insights and opinions is modelling the way staff should seek to empower the person with dementia.

EMPOWERING YOUR STAFF

Empowerment is an important concept in person-centred leadership – supporting staff to take seriously their responsibilities and do their absolute best. It is front-line staff, not dementia care leaders, who have the power to influence the minute-by-minute well-being of people with dementia; what leaders must do is provide a climate where this is most likely to happen.

As I suggested in Chapter 1, person-centred care cannot be delivered solely 'by the book' because its very nature requires staff to be able to respond in the moment to the needs of individuals. This demands much flexibility and resourcefulness on the part of staff, and these qualities need to be cultivated by leaders who encourage creative thinking and enable staff to develop and implement their own ideas, based on the understanding they have developed about the people they are supporting.

This process of empowerment relies on the development of mutual trust between leaders and front-line staff – something which can take some time to grow. On the part of staff, they need to know that they can talk through their ideas and plans and be listened to, and that they can candidly share their experiences – both positive and negative – with a leader who will be prepared to engage in a process of collaborative learning and will certainly not blame them if things have not turned out as they hoped. On the part of the leader, trusting staff to work autonomously means knowing that the staff member shares the same vision and is working towards the same goals as you are.

Harnessing strengths and abilities

Empowering staff means recognising their individual strengths and abilities. In Chapter 1, I illustrated how staff can maximise the potential abilities of people with dementia by working in partnership with them. Empowering staff is also about maximising their potential. Leaders should work in partnership with staff by meeting them at the right point – enabling them fully to use their strengths by providing what they need (see Figure 3.1 for examples). Gaining knowledge of each staff member as an individual is important here – leaders need a clear understanding of each staff member's skills, qualities and talents and the help they require. It is inevitable, within a team of people, that strengths will vary. Some staff, for example, probably have high levels of patience and compassion, while others might be less patient but very energetic and bubbly. Decisions regarding allocations and rotas should always involve consideration of such individual strengths and how these can best be matched to needs of individuals or groups.

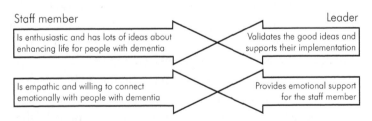

Figure 3.1: Maximising potential of staff through working in partnership

Utilising personal resources

Even the interests and backgrounds of staff can be harnessed to benefit service users.

For example

A staff member who was a keen basketball player put a net in one of the care home lounges and shot hoops as he passed through, encouraging residents to have a go too (Fossey and James 2008).

A staff member who was a keen belly-dancer gave regular demonstrations to residents in the care home where she worked.

Staff who were interested in fashion and make-up led 'beauty therapy' sessions for clients.

Staff who are willing to share aspects of their culture, for example in leading 'theme days'. One Indian care worker had a large collection of saris, which she brought into her care home and helped residents who were interested to try them on.

Who staff members are as people needs to be seen as the key resource they bring to their interactions with people with dementia, and drawing their outside interests into their work clearly confirms that the personhood of staff, as well as the personhood of clients, is appreciated. Being recognised for and encouraged to do something that they love to do anyway is an exhilarating and validating experience for staff, and one that can greatly enhance motivation. Furthermore, their enthusiasm for the pastime is likely to be conveyed to clients, who are then more likely to engage – thus creating a heightened possibility of a successful experience for staff and clients alike.

> What do you know about members of your staff team – their skills and personal qualities; their interests and hobbies; their cultural backgrounds and life experiences?
>
> Which of these personal resources are or could be used in their work with people with dementia? How?

UNDERSTANDING THE FACTORS THAT MOTIVATE YOUR STAFF

It is important to consider what factors motivate people in their work. Person-centred dementia care is both personally and professionally challenging, yet rates of pay do not reflect the high levels of resourcefulness required. The rewards, therefore, need to come from elsewhere, and if dementia care leaders can gain an understanding of the particular motivations of the individuals within their teams, they can seek to maximise these incentives and address any shortfalls before they cause a loss of commitment of the staff member concerned. On the Dementia Care Leadership Programme, candidates use a questionnaire (see the following page) with their teams to analyse the factors that motivate their own staff. This highlights the importance, for example, of staff feeling that they could make suggestions that will be acted on, feeling respected for their efforts and achievements, and feeling part of a team.

Given that dementia care is often challenging and always demanding, staff members who are motivated mainly by the convenience of their workplace and their working hours are unlikely to stay for long if there is any other work available. Staff retention is more likely to come from staff recognising the importance of their own role, finding their work interesting and fulfilling, and having opportunities to develop their skills, confidence and career. These factors will influence staff not only to stay in their jobs but also to do their best, so it is important that leaders are able to motivate and inspire, to show respect for the efforts made by staff and to make it clear that their input is valued.

STAFF MOTIVATIONS QUESTIONNAIRE

This questionnaire asks about the reasons why you are in your current job, and how you feel about it. Please read each statement below and put a tick in one of the four boxes on the right to indicate how true the statement is for you. There are no right or wrong answers and this questionnaire is anonymous.

How well do the following statements describe why you are working in your current job and how you feel about it?	Definitely	Partly	Not very much	Not at all
The hours of the job suit me				
My workplace is convenient for me to get to				
I have always wanted to work with people with dementia				
I enjoy working with older people				
This is not my ideal job, but was the best I could get at the time				
I believe that the work I do is very important				
I can see results for my efforts				
I like my work environment				
I find the job interesting and varied				
I find the job fulfilling				
I get on well with my colleagues				
I would not have chosen to work with people with dementia, but I've now found that I enjoy it				
The work is well-suited to my own abilities and personal qualities				
I feel respected for my efforts and achievements				
The pay and conditions of service are good				
There are good prospects for promotion				
I feel part of a team				
I feel I know everything there is to know about caring for people with dementia				
I feel positive about the organisation I work for				
I have a personal commitment to helping people with dementia experience a good life				

How well do the following statements describe why you are working in your current job and how you feel about it?	Definitely	Partly	Not very much	Not at all
I have strong relationships with many of the people with dementia I care for				
I have good training opportunities and am able to put what I learn into practice				
I am encouraged to use my own ideas in my work				
I like the level of responsibility I have				
I have a vocation for care work				
I feel experienced and confident in my job				
I find people with dementia interesting				
I can make suggestions about how things could be done differently, and these are acted on				
I feel that I am learning all the time from my work				

Now please put a tick in the left hand column against the five most important reasons that describe why you are doing your current job.

Nurturing leadership potential

Through recognising strengths, abilities and positive motivations of staff, managers within dementia care services can also draw out and nurture the leadership potential that exists within the team. Skills and enthusiasm are validated when staff are given the opportunity to become informal leaders through – for example – sharing their experiences, making suggestions, carrying out specific projects or taking on responsibilities like mentoring less experienced or confident staff members. And such team members are allies in the manager's mission to transform the care service.

Managers should look for the kind of team members described by Jerry Sternin (2002) as 'positive deviants' – those who are able to find creative ways forward and solutions to problems that others may have believed could not be solved with the resources available. Sternin says: 'We want to identify these people because they provide demonstrable evidence that solutions to the problem already exist within the community' (Sparks 2004).

For example

A home care worker who, within the same half-hour time slot that others feel is too short to do anything but give personal care to the person with dementia, manages to support the person, by working in partnership, to carry out much of her own personal care.

It will be very beneficial for other home carers and their clients if the manager encourages this staff member to share, at a team meeting, the real-life evidence of how she managed to achieve this.

The creation of more formal leadership roles within the team – such as Dementia Champions – is, as I suggested at the beginning of this book, invaluable for a dementia care service that is serious about moving forward. But it is vital to adequately equip these Dementia Champions to undertake their role if they are to be genuinely empowered to lead from their positions within teams. They need to be given opportunities to develop not only an in-depth understanding of person-centred dementia care, but also skills for guiding and supporting staff – for example the coaching techniques that will be discussed in Chapter 4 of this book. There is a delicate path to tread in attempting to influence practices of colleagues whose jobs are at the same grade as your own. Dementia Champions need a high level of interpersonal skills including tact, persuasion, negotiation and emotional intelligence, but it is also essential that their role is properly recognised within the organisation, so that they are seen by their colleagues to have the right to give advice, ask questions and offer feedback. It is often helpful if organisations establish some formal situations for Dementia Champions to offer guidance including a regular slot within team meetings, a recognised role within care planning and review processes, and some extranumerary hours on a regular basis during which the Dementia Champion can observe, shadow, mentor or even offer some kind of advice surgery.

If Dementia Champion roles are to properly benefit a care service, systems will also need to be established for them to give feedback to managers about changes that might need to be made at an organisational level – adapting the format of care plans, for example, or changing an unhelpful routine that is causing staff to rush and undermine their clients' abilities. The organisation will need to be willing to take such feedback and advice on board, which means it needs to be open to new ideas and prepared to embrace change.

MEETING THE EMOTIONAL NEEDS OF STAFF
Acknowledging feelings

Connecting with the experience of living with dementia can be emotionally disturbing. It is often shocking for staff to realise, for instance, that the vast majority of people with dementia do have some degree of insight into their own difficulties, awareness of what's happening around them, and capacity to experience a full range of human emotion. The myth that people with dementia lack these capabilities has enabled poor care practice to take place without guilt or reproach. Letting go of the myth is painful.

Alongside this emotional challenge, there is also the reality that working with people with dementia is often intense and can be stressful or even frightening. As I will consider in Chapter 6, people with dementia who are experiencing strong feelings and unmet needs can sometimes express themselves in ways that staff find very challenging. If staff are not adequately trained, they are likely to find themselves all the more frequently on the receiving end of 'challenging behaviour', since they are probably inadvertently creating stressful situations for people with dementia and then having to deal with the outcomes.

It is not uncommon for dementia care staff to feel frustrated – for example if they are trying to undertake a task with which their client will not cooperate – or exasperated, as they might if they are having to answer the same question repeatedly. Some staff

> What feelings have you noticed or heard staff expressing recently?
>
> How do you think these feelings have affected their work?

might find it exhausting to constantly have to think on their feet, for instance to try to divert a resident who is determined to get out of the care home because she is convinced that she has to collect her children from school. And working closely with people who are experiencing strong emotions can sometimes trigger the emotions of staff, particularly if a person is reliving painful memories that resonate with something the staff member themselves has been through. These feelings can easily impact on the staff member's approach.

Supporting staff with their feelings

There is a strong equation between the kind of support that staff receive and the kind of support they give to the people they care for. If dementia care staff do not receive sufficient support, they generally find that the only way to manage their own feelings is to construct a defensive barrier between themselves and those they care for. This creates an emotional disconnection that blocks empathy and inhibits relationships. But when leaders attend to the emotional needs of staff and work at developing trusting relationships with them, they are both modelling exactly how they want staff to be with the people they care for, and also making it safe for staff to draw on their own emotions and humanity to develop and sustain truly person-centred relationships with people with dementia.

Just as good dementia care involves connecting with the reality of living with dementia, good dementia care leadership involves a deep understanding of the reality of working with people with dementia. Leaders must acknowledge the feelings expressed by staff about their work, even in situations where you might have a strong suspicion that the staff member has created stress for their client and for themselves by approaching a situation badly. It is important to recognise positive intentions, even if these are misguided; to believe in a staff member's potential to improve their approach if they are given the right help.

Providing one-to-one support

One of the most important ways for leaders to provide this emotional support is simply by making it clear that you are there for staff when they need you, and you are willing to listen. When a member of staff has been finding

> How do you indicate your interest and concern?
>
> How do you respond when staff express their feelings?

their work difficult, being able to express their own feelings to a supportive leader who really listens and does not judge is extremely helpful. Active listening involves focusing fully on the other person and putting your own thoughts and concerns aside for a while. Sometimes you don't need to say anything, but just show through your body language and facial expression that you are listening. At other times it might be helpful to indicate your understanding and empathy by reflecting back or paraphrasing what the staff member is saying and what they seem to be communicating non-verbally. Through having an opportunity to offload, and feeling understood, the staff member's own capacity for empathic understanding will be revitalised. And sometimes, through having the opportunity to talk through their problems, staff muster their own insight and creativity to find a constructive way forward. Through active listening, you are communicating not only your support, but also your belief that the person's thoughts and feelings are valuable. As Nicholas Iuppa (1986, p.69) said: 'Just being available and attentive is a great way to use listening as a management tool. Some employees will come in, talk for twenty minutes, and leave having solved their problems entirely by themselves.'

When staff are experiencing personal problems that don't relate to their work, it is important for the sake of your relationship with the staff member that you show some interest and concern, though of course it is not required – or appropriate – that you provide personal counselling to each member of your team. However, it is important to recognise when a person's own problems are distracting them to such an extent that they don't have sufficient attention for their work. If possible, you may need to rearrange rotas so that the person can take some leave, or perhaps there is scope to temporarily shift the person within the organisation to a less stressful area of work. It's very useful if you are aware of services that provide employee counselling so that you can refer the staff member to sources of further help.

In group care settings there will be frequent opportunities for informal contact with staff – brief chats during which you can gain a sense of the staff member's state of mind and catch up on what's going on with the people with dementia they're supporting. The more you know each staff member, the easier it will be to judge what the person needs.

For example

One leader found that by knowing her staff well she was able to pick up when things didn't appear to be going well for them. Simply by saying 'Are you OK?' or 'You know where I am if you need me', she made staff aware that she wanted to support them.

In a home care setting or any other community-based service, much of your contact with staff will take place over the phone; it's important that you are available to listen to concerns that staff need to share, and indeed that they are encouraged to make contact when they need support. It's all too easy to slip into a focus on practicalities and to lose sight of emotions, but such a situation will quickly lead to a task-focused approach to care. Being constantly mindful of feelings when talking with staff about their work is an important example to set.

In more formal one-to-one situations, such as supervision and appraisal sessions, the focus on feelings is also important. While there are certain procedural requirements in terms of issues that need to be addressed in such meetings, it is important for both parties that they are seen as constructive developmental opportunities – a chance for the staff member to reflect on their practice, develop and share ideas and receive constructive feedback. And attention must also be paid to the staff member's emotional well-being – here is a key opportunity for them to receive your full attention while they express their feelings about their work – to be encouraged, for example, to talk about what they've been finding hard, what successes they are proud of, and how their relationships with their clients are progressing.

Offering group support

Team meetings should also provide opportunities for staff to talk about the realities of their day-to-day work and feel supported in doing so. Facing and meeting the challenges of dementia care can be a hugely rewarding experience for a staff team that works together supportively and cooperatively. Group discussions can offer valuable opportunities for collaborative enquiry and discovery – for example pooling ideas to find ways forward that individuals have not been able to discover on their own. Skilful leadership is important to draw out such creative thinking and maintain an optimistic focus. Team discussions can easily degenerate into collusive grumbling sessions where problems, rather than potential solutions, receive the group's attention; leaders need to steer discussions away from generalisations and assumptions and keep focused on individuals and their potential for enhanced well-being. Some strategies for problem-solving in teams are explored in Chapter 6.

Establishing staff-led peer support groups can also be a beneficial way of fostering positive relationships within the team and enabling people to offload some of their feelings, as long as there are clear ground rules that ensure everyone has an equal opportunity to participate and the group steers away from a problem-centred focus. The use of structured listening techniques – such as each person having five minutes to talk about what's going well and what's difficult – can encourage people to listen properly to each other and support a positive focus.

MANAGING TEAM DYNAMICS

The productivity of team meetings and peer support groups will also depend on relationships between individuals and the group dynamics within the staff team. Various factors influence the process by which people interact and behave in teams including, for example, the personalities of individuals, the diversity of team members, and the differing levels of skill, experience and commitment. It is easy for cliques to develop and for individuals to slip into particular negative roles that detract from the team's overall performance – for example someone might become the team's 'joker'; another staff member might be the one who always tends to dominate meetings and discussions. Leaders may have to work hard to try to break up cliques and manage disruptive behaviours, for instance by giving people separate responsibilities according to their individual strengths, and pairing up individuals who might not normally choose to work together. The style of your leadership has a big influence on the types of relationships that develop within the team. An open and inclusive style of leadership, for example, will increase the likelihood of a mutually respectful climate within the group; a leader who listens well not only role models but also encourages good listening among group members. It is important for the team dynamics that the leader is seen to notice and champion good practice, and also to quickly identify and address poor practice: this reduces the likelihood of a culture of complaining and scapegoating developing.

One key role of the leader in building a cooperative team is to help members see how every individual plays a part in the team's work and influences its outcomes. Everything that each team member does (or doesn't do) impacts on everyone else, so a single action creates ripples that may extend way beyond the individual's immediate awareness.

For example

A staff member in the day centre thoughtlessly criticises a person with dementia for making a mess at the dining table... The person with dementia feels angry and upset; this festers for a while until another service user accidentally knocks over her walking stick and the anger spills out as a verbally abusive outburst... The mood within the day centre is affected; various people, upset by the incident, feel unsettled and ask to go home... The afternoon's activities fall flat, and the staff who have carefully planned them feel demoralised...

Clearly negative actions can have far-reaching effects but, crucially, positive ones can too. The reality is that anybody can make a positive difference from any place in the organisation.

For example

A domestic worker has a warm and humorous chat with a person with dementia... The person's mood improves and he is still feeling happy when his son visits later in the afternoon... The son is hugely encouraged to see his dad with a smile on his face – he had been feeling very guilty about his dad moving into residential care but now he starts to feel a bit more optimistic about the future...

Leaders can help staff become aware of the positive knock-on effects of their actions by highlighting positive evidence and discovering with their team – for example at a handover meeting – how these outcomes came about. This is a really important process in helping staff become aware of their own power to influence the well-being of the people with dementia with whom they come into contact. Where outcomes have been negative (as in the first example above) a similar process of analysis is important but care must be taken not to publicly blame individuals for the adverse results of their actions. A process of constructive feedback (to be described in Chapter 4) will be much more likely to bring about insight and improvement.

Successful teamwork depends on mutually respectful relationships where each team member understands their role and contribution to the group and is valued for the part they play. Having shared priorities helps to increase trust within a staff team and will contribute to a spirit of cooperation across different shifts of staff and different job roles within the team. Person-centred leaders value every positive contribution and empower each team member to make a positive impact.

Table 3.1 Chapter 3 key points

Key points	What leaders need to do
Leaders should be role models for person-centred care	Be involved with clients; be seen to do everything that staff should do, with the approach you would wish them to adopt
Empowerment is integral to person-centred leadership	Ensure that staff are equipped for their role and encourage them to use their strengths
High levels of motivation are needed for person-centred dementia care	Gain an understanding of what motivates individuals; respect and value their work and their ideas
Changing a culture of care requires leaders from within the team as well as at its helm	Search for leadership potential within teams and empower new leaders to take on specific responsibilities
Person-centred care needs the emotional involvement of staff	Provide emotional support for staff through attentive listening, showing empathy and giving time
Cooperative teamwork is key to person-centred dementia care	Model respectful communication; highlight the impact of individuals' contributions

Chapter 4

Creating a Learning Culture

The Role of Training and Reflective Practice

By the end of this chapter, you will:

- Have considered how to get the best outcomes from training.
- Have thought about observation as a useful learning tool.
- Recognise the importance of helping staff learn from their own experiences.
- Know how to facilitate reflective practice through questioning feedback and constructive response to bad practice.

Person-centred care is possible only through learning about individuals, and the needs of these individuals will change continuously. Therefore a dementia care service that aims to be person-centred must develop a learning culture. This involves the provision not only of excellent training but also – even more importantly – of on-the-job coaching to support learning from experience.

GETTING THE BEST OUT OF TRAINING
Finding the right training

Dementia training is now more firmly on the national agenda than in previous times, prompted by the National Dementia Strategy recommendation for 'An informed and effective workforce for people with dementia' (Department of Health 2009). A comprehensive induction programme is essential for new recruits, and, as staff develop more experience, further training will be required to address emerging needs. Training is equally important for long-standing staff, to help refresh their knowledge and practice, develop new skills and increase motivation. However, it is very important to be aware that only part of the necessary learning can be achieved in a classroom, and only then if staff are attending a training course that is specifically geared to their needs and concerns.

Too often, training is seen as an end in itself – the assumption is that a manager can send a staff member on a course and they will return to work able to do their job better. What's important, though, is not that staff are exposed to training, but that they actually learn from it. It's perfectly possible to attend a training course and come away none the wiser, particularly if staff are not motivated to learn because they feel that what they are being taught is not necessary or relevant to their work. It needs to be acknowledged that for many more experienced staff, being faced with new ideas actually feels quite threatening, since there is an inherent implication that the way they have been doing things over the years might not be the best way.

In order to support participants to actually learn, training needs to involve much more than just the imparting of information. Relatively few people learn well from sitting and listening to lectures; it is important that the training is engaging, addresses different learning styles and provides practical guidance on how staff can put what they are learning into practice. The course needs to be pitched at an appropriate level, building on knowledge that participants already have, while addressing gaps.

There are some training needs that are likely to exist in any dementia care service, for example learning what dementia actually is and what it means to live with the condition and 'unlearning' the commonly held mistaken beliefs and misinformation that I identified in Chapter 2. Little use is served by training courses that focus only on factual information about dementia; staff also need guidance on how to support people who have it, which surely is the most important matter. It is also important that some kind of training needs analysis has been carried out to identify the requirements of the individuals who will be attending a course: in this way the most appropriate training can be commissioned and the course can focus on participants' areas of concern and enable them to feel that their requests are being addressed.

Supporting the implementation of new learning

Training cannot, on its own, transform attitudes and practices. Leaders within the care setting have a key role to play after the training course in enabling staff to consolidate their insights and put into practice what they have learnt. The starting point is simply to show interest – encourage the person to talk through their new learning and develop their thoughts on some of the things they are intending to do differently as a result. It will often be useful to talk about specifics, such as how the staff member might try out their newly learnt communication techniques with one particular service user who currently seems very withdrawn. Ask the staff

> Consider the dementia training that your staff attend. Is it sufficient? What have been the key learning points? Do these influence attitudes and practice? Is there more that you could do to help staff implement their learning? Are there changes that need to be made to the training itself in order to improve the outcomes?

member to share any new ideas they have as a result of their training. For example, if someone has been on a course about occupations and activities, encourage them to take the lead in setting up a new activity for clients. Be prepared to help the person access the resources they might need, while empowering them to take the lead.

Above all else, staff will benefit from training only if it is just one component in a wider strategy of development, rooted in a consistent philosophy that is reflected throughout the care service. If a staff member returns from their training course and sees, for example, that the dementia care leaders in their workplace are implementing the very same approach that they have just been learning about, their new learning will be consolidated. If this is not what they witness, any new learning will quickly be lost.

Formal training may be important, but alongside this, workplace-based learning is essential. This means that dementia care leaders have a key role in guiding, coaching and role modelling, facilitating the most important kind of learning of all for person-centred dementia care: learning through experiences.

DEVELOPING OBSERVATIONAL SKILLS OF STAFF

Observation can be an important way of learning through experiences. I have already suggested that when staff are involved in observing individuals' well-being, they can become more aware of people's needs, see behaviour in a different light, and notice the positive and negative effects of their work with individuals. Other kinds of observation can also be useful learning activities for staff to undertake. It is easy for busy staff to make assumptions and lose sight of details. Offering each staff member, on a regular basis, a half-hour time period when they are relieved of their normal duties and asked, instead, to observe can be a great way of prompting them to notice and reflect on the things they have been overlooking.

Observations could focus on a general area, a particular concern, or even a specific person. What is important is that the parameters are established before the observation takes place and the staff member sets out with some idea about what they're looking for.

For example

A staff member could be asked to spend time focusing on a group of people in the lounge, looking for any signs of boredom, and noticing anything that clients were actively involved in doing.

They could be asked to observe the general atmosphere at lunchtime, paying particular attention to noise levels.

They could be asked to observe one specific person with dementia, trying to discover something in particular – is there any indication that Muriel is in pain, for example, or otherwise becoming distressed, and what are the factors that precipitate this?

This last example could be particularly useful for a staff member who is inclined to jump too quickly to conclusions, or for a staff team who are struggling to understand the reasons for Muriel's sudden outbursts of angry words. It also helps to remind the staff member that being attentive to non-verbal communication is always important as a way of understanding the needs of people with dementia.

It is clear that spending time observing can prompt insights that would not occur in the general course of everyday work. Importantly, any such observation needs to be immediately followed by a debriefing session to talk about what was noticed and draw out insights. And thought needs to be given to what the individual will do with their insights – how these will be fed back to the team in an acceptable way (ensuring that the individual is not interpreted as criticising their colleagues) and when this will happen.

HELPING STAFF REFLECT ON THEIR PRACTICE

The debriefing session after an observation is a vital part of the learning process. It is often said that the best learning comes from our experiences; we are all familiar, for example, with the concept of learning from mistakes. But, as Arin-Krupp (cited in York-Barr, Sommers and Ghere 2006) reminds us, 'adults do not learn from experience, they learn from processing experience'. In other words, we have to think about experiences we have in order to learn from them. Without doing so, we're no further forward than we were before the experience, and we are liable to carry on making the same mistakes.

Reflective practice – thinking about and learning from what you're doing – is central to person-centred dementia care. Once we understand that each person with dementia is an individual, with unique needs, we are led to the inevitable conclusion that there is no single way of providing care. All the guidelines in the world could not tell us about Dorothy, who has just moved into the care home. We have to get to know her for ourselves and learn from each interaction we have with her; each piece of information shared by others who know her.

The process of reflective practice can be described (for example by Kolb 1983) as a cycle involving four stages, each of which leads on to the next (see also Figure 4.1):

1. You have an experience.

2. You reflect on the experience.

3. You draw conclusions and learn from the experience.

4. You decide how to use your learning and plan your next steps.

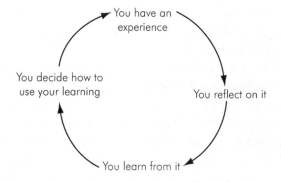

You have an
experience

You decide how to
use your learning

You reflect on it

You learn from it

Figure 4.1: The learning cycle (adapted from Kolb 1983)

For example

You have an experience:

Having a conversation with Dorothy about her personal care needs. She talks about feeling very embarrassed because she needs some help with washing.

You reflect on the experience:

Thinking about what it is in particular that causes embarrassment for Dorothy and how to minimise her embarrassment while helping her wash.

You draw conclusions and learn from the experience:

Realising that the key issue for Dorothy is that she doesn't want to expose her body, particularly since she doesn't yet know any of the care staff very well.

You decide how to use your learning and plan your next steps:

Deciding to spend a little time chatting to Dorothy each morning before offering personal care so that she can gradually get to know the care staff better. Ensuring that Dorothy's bath towel is large enough to keep her covered at all times while she is being helped to wash so that she can retain maximum privacy and dignity.

The next step – where we have returned to the 'having an experience' stage of the learning cycle – is an opportunity to put the plan into action.

The above example of Dorothy's personal care is provided as a straightforward illustration of the use of the learning cycle in person-centred care provision. It represents a simple situation in which any but the most oblivious staff member would be prompted to take on board what the person with dementia has said and work out how to accommodate her wishes.

In real life, however, many situations are less simple. Specifically, a key complicating factor is that dementia often impacts on communication abilities, so understanding Dorothy's embarrassment is likely to require more of the care worker than just listening to what she says.

For example

Dorothy might communicate her embarrassment by refusing to cooperate. Perhaps she is very reluctant to get out of bed and accompany the care worker to the bathroom. If she does go into the bathroom, she might be unwilling to remove her nightclothes. She might non-verbally express that she is unhappy through her facial expression and body language; she might make distressed noises. If the care worker (concerned, perhaps, to achieve the personal care task that is her responsibility) tries to insist – and perhaps starts to remove Dorothy's nightclothes anyway – she may well scream, attempt to push the care worker away, or lash out.

Clearly Dorothy's message, in this situation, is exactly the same as her message in the first example: 'I am embarrassed to be helped to wash and I don't want to be exposed.' The only thing that's different is Dorothy's communication ability. But a common problem in this kind of situation is that the person's message is not understood. As Graham Stokes (2008) writes, typically there is no attempt made to understand the reason for the person's reaction, because this reaction is experienced by staff as challenging, and the 'challenging behaviour' is then assumed to be a symptom of their dementia. So, as Stokes says, no-one tries to discover the reason because the reason is believed to be blatantly obvious: 'It is because they have dementia.'

As we saw in Chapter 2, we have been plagued by misinformation and unhelpful beliefs about dementia, and if these are brought to bear in reflecting on an experience such as the incident with Dorothy, the learning cycle becomes blocked or diverted at the 'reflecting' stage of the process, hitting a brick wall rather than continuing round (see Figure 4.2).

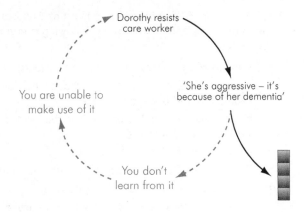

Figure 4.2: The blocked learning cycle

In this situation, useful conclusions cannot be drawn, nor can plans for future action be formulated. If 'it's the dementia' is the reflection, then what could be concluded but 'isn't dementia terrible?' It is a vital role of dementia care leaders to support the process of reflective practice, ensuring that the cycle does not get rerouted down such an unhelpful track.

In the subsequent sections of this chapter I will examine some of the ways in which leaders can facilitate reflective practice.

Using questions to guide reflective practice

One of the key ways in which leaders can help staff develop their reflective practice is by asking questions to prompt the processes of reflecting, concluding and planning. The questions might be quite open, simply encouraging a staff member to share their thoughts on a situation. Or the leader might need to ask specific questions that will help the staff member realise what assumptions she might have been making and what she could do differently the next time.

For example

To support the care worker to reflect on Dorothy's refusal to engage in personal care, some of the following questions might be helpful:

- Why do you think Dorothy wouldn't cooperate?
- What was she communicating through her facial expression and body language?
- How would you feel if you had to be helped to wash by a care worker?
- How do you think Dorothy was feeling?
- Do you think Dorothy understood who you were?
- Did she know what you were trying to do?
- Is there anything extra you could have done to help her understand?
- What's your relationship with Dorothy like?
- Do you think she trusts you?
- How could you build a closer relationship and help her trust you more?
- What could you do to help Dorothy feel less embarrassed?

The outcome of these questions should, I hope, be a heightened awareness on the part of the care worker of Dorothy's feelings and needs and how these can be addressed.

Now it may well be that the leader already knows or guesses the answers to some or all of these questions. Indeed, when the staff member comes to report that 'Dorothy kicked off again', you may feel that it would be quicker and simpler to bypass the questions and share your own reflections and conclusion with the care worker: 'Dorothy was obviously feeling embarrassed and was uncertain about what was happening. You need to get to know her better, explain what you're doing and provide a larger bath towel.'

But while there are some situations where giving advice might be the most helpful way forward, there are two problems with this strategy. First, leaders don't usually have all the answers. Front-line staff are likely to have more contact with and a deeper knowledge of the individuals they're supporting,

> Think about the difference between being told something and discovering something for yourself.
>
> Which learning is more powerful? Which is more memorable?

so finding the best way forward often genuinely requires the staff member's input. If you give advice, it might not be based on a full understanding of the person or the situation, and therefore might be neither helpful nor applicable. Second, giving answers rather than asking for them is quite simply less effective. Perhaps the staff member will remember to act on your advice the next time, but it's just as likely that she won't. She might not agree with your recommendation; perhaps she doesn't fully understand it, or she may quite simply forget what you've suggested as the old habits take over. If she does act on your advice, and if her personal care task with Dorothy goes more smoothly as a result, let's hope that she'll learn from this experience and may then continue with her improved practice. But if Dorothy's response isn't immediately different as a result of her adapted approach, she's quite likely to revert to her old practices. This is because the staff member hasn't personally engaged in the processes of reflection and conclusion and therefore has no real investment in the plans.

Far more learning is generated if staff are helped to work things out for themselves. It may take them longer to reach the conclusion that you've already reached, but they are far more likely to remember it, act on it, and be committed to the way forward that they have mapped out for themselves. Through asking the right questions, you can prompt the staff member to look beneath the surface, to develop empathy, to understand the meaning communicated through behaviour, and to develop their understanding of an individual and his or her needs. They may even learn some general principles that could be applied more widely, in different contexts and with different people. It is important that a question is not phrased in a way that will make the staff member feel defensive. 'Why did you…', for example, is an opening to be avoided – it's more of an accusation than a question that could help the person learn. Questions should not be designed to highlight mistakes or weaknesses, but to facilitate learning through suggesting areas for the staff member to consider. And once the person has gained some insight, prompting them to talk about how they will make use of this is very important. When people express their thoughts out loud, and are listened to, they are much more likely to act on their intentions and put their plans into action.

Coaching staff through the learning cycle, or 'reflecting-*on*-action' (Schön 1987) also enables them to begin thinking on their feet so that they can be more responsive in the moment – developing the ability to 'reflect-*in*-action'. This is essential if staff are to meet the complex and ever-changing needs of people with dementia. Being sensitive, responsive and flexible are integral to person-centred care, and all require the ability to 'reflect-in-action'.

Giving feedback

I have met many leaders within dementia care who are passionate about wanting things to be better for people with dementia in their own care service; who despair at the poor attitudes and task-focused mentality they encounter from a minority – or even a majority – of their staff group and who are determined to address poor practices. They are to be commended for their fire and determination, without which things would never shift. However, what's crucial is that their passion is channelled into strategies that will bring about real and lasting change. However much passion a leader has, no-one can single-handedly change a culture of care. The way to change things in an organisation is through bringing people with you.

So when you become aware of an area of practice that needs to change it is important to think about how this could most helpfully be communicated. Telling staff what they have done wrong, and perhaps telling them off for it, is tempting. Indeed, this is a natural reaction when you feel strongly about the bad practice you have witnessed. But unfortunately reproach will be unlikely to motivate changes for the better. It is more probable that staff in receipt of such criticism will feel angry or disheartened. They may become quite defensive, seeking to present reasons or excuses for their actions. Their opinion of their critic (you) may decline, in which case they will mentally dismiss what they've been told. At best, they may learn what not to do when they are being watched. Clearly this is unlikely to improve their practice more widely.

Validation

In order to enable staff to recognise and learn from their mistakes, we must (counter-intuitive though it may seem) be prepared to help them learn about their successes. People learn much more from being told what they have done right than from hearing what they have done wrong. A staff member who is validated by their manager for a positive action is very likely to repeat the same action, whereas someone who has been told off for doing something wrong will tend simply to feel disgruntled. In fact, validation is essential in order to build and maintain a positive approach – without validation, good practice will gradually wither and die.

I hope that all leaders reading this book will be able to think of recent occasions when you have praised or thanked members of your staff group. This might have taken place in a formal situation, such as a supervision session or a performance and development review. Or in some kind of impromptu situation, where you might have shown your appreciation of a staff member for doing more than was expected of them – a care worker who stayed on after his shift had finished, because he was comforting a resident who had been upset; a home care worker who visited one of her clients in hospital on her day off; a day centre worker who set up a new activity that all the clients are enjoying. Such practices certainly do deserve lots of validation!

But how often have you praised staff for doing exactly what they should be doing? A care worker who is chatting pleasantly to a resident while walking with her to the dining room, for example. Would you offer a few words of validation after the event? Possibly not, because after all someone simply doing their job properly is not an 'event' that would be likely to attract anything more than your passing attention. But if you do commend this kind of everyday good practice, it will increase the probability that the care worker will chat to the resident again the next time she escorts her. And she'll be more likely to chat to other residents

Do you always comment when a staff member has done something well? Are you more likely to comment when they have done something wrong? Can you think of any recent examples of good practice that you've noticed but not mentioned?

too, and other staff may follow her example. Thus the seeds of good practice are watered and fertilised.

The most helpful form of validation involves more than simply saying 'thank-you'. Not that there's anything wrong with offering thanks – in fact it is essential to do so to help staff feel appreciated and so to keep up their morale. But more descriptive and specific validation not only helps staff feel valued, but also helps them learn what they have done that has been particularly valuable and gain confidence in their own skills. So validation confirms and establishes good practice by clarifying standards and expectations.

Using this strategy could be a matter simply of praising a specific interaction that you witnessed between a staff member and a client: 'Well done for being so patient when you were helping Mary eat her lunch', for example. Or even just letting the staff member know that you have noticed their efforts: 'You were really patient with Mary at lunch.' Some staff will brush off such comments as if they are unnecessary, but don't be fooled; no-one genuinely dislikes positive feedback, even if some people may feel a little embarrassed by it. This is probably indicative of the fact that the person hasn't received enough positive feedback in their life. It's important, though, that validation is offered in a way that doesn't feel patronising or sarcastic.

It is most helpful if validation is as specific as possible rather than fluffy, generalised comments such as 'that was a good interaction'. Depending on the nature of the good practice you have observed, you might be able to make detailed comments about what the staff member did well. It will be very useful to do so.

For example

'I heard you speaking in a really gentle tone of voice to George earlier…that was so helpful to him because he'd been feeling very anxious all morning. I noticed that after you'd spent that time with him he was much calmer and happier.'

'I saw that when you were helping Joyce put her coat on, you really gave her the opportunity to do everything she could for herself...you just showed her where the top buttonhole was, didn't you? And then she managed to do all the buttons up for herself. That's something really important you helped her achieve.'

'It's great that you stopped and listened to Margaret when she starting speaking to you on the corridor earlier on. I know you were in a hurry, but you were really careful that you didn't make her feel unimportant. In fact you only spent about 20 seconds with her, but she walked away smiling to herself!'

Making positive comments about a staff member's approach is one of the quickest and easiest ways to give validation. There are other ways of validating good practice too – for example, speaking about it at a staff meeting, writing about it in a newsletter or asking a staff member who has done something well to teach or support others who are trying to do it too.

Do not underestimate the importance of the validation of good practice in establishing and maintaining a positive culture of care. It should be something that happens all the time and ideally it should come from peers as well as managers. In a positive culture of care, there are always good practices happening that should be commented on. If such comments don't come naturally at first, it's really worth practising, until validation becomes second nature.

Validation can also play a key role in improving care practice. Let's imagine an area of poor practice against which you're continually battling. It might be something you've mentioned a number of times to staff, but improvements are not taking place quickly enough.

For example

Perhaps staff are in the habit of remaining standing when they are talking to people who are sitting down. Despite your prompts and reminders, many of the staff frequently forget to get down to the person's level when communicating; only infrequently do you witness it happening.

So these latter examples are exactly the occasions that you must look for and validate. This isn't to say that you shouldn't carry on reminding staff about what they should be doing on occasions when they're not doing it, but this would be pointless unless you also comment positively when you do see the practice that you want.

It's easier to feed back on good practice when you've seen something happening with your own eyes. But in some care situations, this rarely happens. For example, dementia care leaders within a home care service won't be able to achieve the same view of care practices that those working in a group care setting will naturally have. On any occasion when practice is observed it will be essential to offer full and constructive feedback to the home care worker, and all feedback received from service users, their families and other professionals should be shared with the staff member.

Constructive feedback

So whenever feedback is given, validation should be part of it. But when mistakes have been made, these also need to be mentioned and it is important to think about how this should best be done. As mentioned earlier, when staff feel undermined they are likely to become defensive. In truth, there's not much point in simply telling people what they have done wrong – even in a disciplinary situation – because at best we are teaching them what not to do, but this doesn't offer any guidance as to what should be done in its place. Bearing in mind the aim of developing a learning culture, where reflective practice is the norm, it is essential to support staff in the process of learning from all aspects of their practice – mistakes as well as successes. The starting point of this – as with every other aspect of good practice – is the leader as a role model. In terms of learning from experience, leaders need to be open about their mistakes – to be prepared to admit what they have got wrong, to ask staff for advice about what they could have done better, and to be clear that they don't 'know it all'. Webb (1995) explains that reflective practice requires openness, letting go of the need to be right.

A useful and memorable model for constructive feedback is 'www.ebi' – which stands for *w*hat *w*ent *w*ell and *e*ven *b*etter *i*f. However well we have done something, it's likely that there are ways in which we can improve further on our practice. When every aspect of the person's good practice has been validated and we have ensured that the person receiving the feedback has taken in the information about what they've done well, these positive practices can then serve as the scaffolding from which the person can be supported to build still further on their skills. The use of 'www.ebi' could go as follows:

For example

You notice a staff member walking around the garden with two residents, both of whom have dementia. She is between them, linking arms with them both, and walking slowly. One of the residents is very talkative and the staff member is engaging well with her as they walk. The other resident is quiet (she is often withdrawn), though she appears to be enjoying looking at the flowers in the garden. Throughout the ten-minute walk in the garden, the staff member's attention is focused on the chatty resident, looking around and smiling at the other lady only once in a while.

After the staff member returns inside and settles both the residents back in the lounge, you ask if you could have a brief word with her, during which you say something such as:

'That was a great idea to take Radhika and Sarah for a walk around the garden. You were walking at their pace and giving them both lovely smiles. The way you linked arms with both of them looked really affectionate and sociable as well. It looked like you were really listening to Radhika and engaging with her. I wonder if Sarah might have felt a bit left out, though? It would be even better if you could find a way of helping her join in the conversation too, or perhaps sharing more of your attention with her. I think she responds really well to you and if anyone can draw her out, then you can.'

The aim of constructive feedback is to help people become more effective. It provides a vital component in the ongoing process of staff development and can influence positive changes. But it will achieve these aims only if it is fair, balanced and non-judgemental. It must be accurate, trying to avoid adverbs of frequency such as 'never' or 'always' and other such hasty generalisations. And it needs to be delivered in a way that enables people to hear it and take it on board. It should never be used as an opportunity to vent feelings or make the person feel small, however angry the leader is, because this will quite simply block the possibility of improvement.

Sometimes it is useful to try to begin and end the feedback on a positive note, because if you start off negatively you risk sabotaging the possibility of the person listening properly at all, and if you finish negatively, the person easily forgets the positive feedback you gave. As we considered earlier, people tend to learn most from hearing what they have done right, even if their good practice was the smaller part of what they did, so it's vital that this information doesn't get lost. This method of giving feedback is sometimes known as a 'feedback sandwich'. It is important not to overuse this format, though, because the staff member will just be waiting for the 'negative bit' in the middle and therefore will not hear anything else. Most helpful of all is when the giving of feedback becomes a regular and expected role of the leader, and this feedback consists primarily of validation.

The 'even better if…' component of the feedback must be based on positive regard and a belief that the person has the potential to get it right. It may be that the receiver of the feedback needs further training or guidance to achieve what is required; the staff member can only work within their own capabilities, with the level of understanding and skills they currently have. It will be counterproductive to make suggestions that are idealistic rather than practical. It's also important that we are considerate of the feelings and responses of the person who is receiving our feedback: there will only be so much that the person is able to absorb, and to carry on beyond that point would be to risk wiping out what they have already learnt from us.

Dealing with bad practice

Giving constructive feedback is clearly not an appropriate strategy for every shortfall. At times, a leader may need to take decisive action. When a person with dementia is being abused or put at risk because of a staff member's poor practice or negligence, the leader has no option but to be directive, taking whatever action is necessary to protect the service user. Every care service should have a disciplinary procedure. This helps to protect clients from abuse, but it should also be seen as a tool to promote staff development, through helping people understand the seriousness of their actions or inactions and setting targets and ultimatums. Staff need to be offered the support and training necessary to enable them to fulfil requirements that have been set, and their progress closely monitored. Ultimately, if they are unable or unwilling to improve their practice – if no amount of training, guidance or constructive feedback makes a positive difference – it is not appropriate that the person should continue working with vulnerable people. But for some staff, disciplinary proceedings are the catalyst for turning around their practice.

There are many situations we may encounter where a staff member's practice is far from good, but their bad practice is not a disciplinary matter. The staff member has disempowered or upset a person with dementia, for instance, through their unthinking and hurried approach. In such situations the thought of providing any positive feedback would seem like a ludicrous idea. But even in this kind of situation, if at all possible we need to find something to validate otherwise there is a real risk that the person's practice could deteriorate still further. Let's consider the following situation:

For example

Carla, a day centre worker, is sitting at the table with a client – Clive, helping him eat lunch, or rather, to be blunt, feeding him – because although Clive is able to eat by himself if his cutlery is placed in his hands and he is given verbal prompts, Carla is doing none of this. She is shovelling food onto the fork and into his mouth. She waits, silently, for him to finish each mouthful, and then shovels more food in. In fact 'silently' isn't quite an accurate description either, because every so often she chats briefly to another staff member sitting at the next table.

Clearly this is far from the approach you want to see and there are many aspects of Carla's practice that are unsatisfactory. Of course you could call her aside and give her a dressing down – you could reel off a list of aspects of her practice that she must improve and set a timescale for improvement. You might feel that this is exactly what she needs; certainly it's the very least she deserves if she knows that this is not acceptable practice. But here's the conundrum: if she actually needs this information, it means she doesn't already know it and therefore she doesn't deserve to be told off for not acting on it. In other words, she doesn't know how else she could help Clive to eat. In fact, if she's never had this information, it's completely unfair to tell her off for her unwitting bad practice; rather, she needs an apology for her lack of induction training and an immediate relocation to an office job until her training needs can be addressed.

But the truth is that Carla probably does already know the difference between good practice and bad practice, because her manager has gone over and over this until she's blue in the face. So why isn't Carla already behaving differently? We talked earlier about the learning cycle – the need to review experiences in order to learn from them. So what conclusions might be drawn by Carla's manager if she reflects on all the times she has explained how to support clients at mealtimes and told staff off when they do not adhere to these guidelines? Perhaps she would conclude that if she actually wants things to change, it might be worth trying a different approach.

If Carla's manager is going to implement the 'www.ebi' model, she first needs to find the 'what went well' component. On first consideration it may seem that this doesn't exist, but in truth, unless a misdemeanour is such that it warrants summary dismissal, then there are always some saving graces, however minor. In Carla's case there are a number of things she did right:

> What 'saving graces' can you find in poor practice you witness? If there's anything at all that the staff member is doing right, it's important to validate it before it disappears altogether.

For example

1. She sat down.
2. She stayed with one client throughout the meal.
3. She waited until he had finished one mouthful before offering another.
4. Although she spoke to another staff member, this was only briefly, and not in any disparaging terms

about the client she was with (although it's a little dubious whether not doing an even worse thing constitutes doing something right! But it is a saving grace, nevertheless).

Constructive feedback, then, could take the following shape:

For example

'I was really pleased to see that you stayed with Clive for the whole of lunch today. And it was good that you were sitting down – being on the same level as someone you're helping conveys respect. I think you could show Clive even more respect if you give him more of an opportunity to use his own abilities next time – help him to pick up his cutlery and then all he'll need are some gentle verbal prompts. Try to keep focused on him – instead of talking to your colleague, you could try chatting to Clive about cricket. It might take a little longer but I know you're really patient by the way I saw you make sure you waited until he'd swallowed before you offered him more... Let me know how it goes...'

CONCLUSION

Every person who works within a care setting or service contributes to the quality of life of individuals receiving care. Every interaction – or lack of interaction – makes an impact of some kind on people with dementia, from the warm glow generated by a sincere smile to the sense of loneliness experienced by someone who is ignored by a passing staff member. No dementia care leader will be present during every moment of contact between staff and people with dementia, and therefore leading positive changes means influencing the attitudes and motivation that internally guide each staff member – growing their capacity for reflective practice and enabling their learning and development.

Table 4.1 Chapter 4 key points

Key points	What leaders need to do
Training is not an end in itself	Ensure that the content and training methods are led by the needs of participants; support people to implement their new learning
Observation can help to prompt awareness and learning	Create opportunities for staff to spend time observing
The process of learning involves experiencing, reflecting, concluding and planning	Help staff progress through the stages of learning from their experiences
Questions can help staff develop their own capacity for reflection	Ask helpful questions that prompt staff to look beneath the surface and develop their empathic awareness
Without validation, good practice will wither and die	Notice and comment on good practice, including everyday aspects of good practice
Constructive feedback can help people become more effective	Sensitively and respectfully tell people what – specifically – they have done well and what they could do even better

Chapter 5

Ensuring Effective Communication with Staff, Families and Professionals

By the end of this chapter, you will:

- Know how to create care plans that guide person-centred care.

- Have considered how to maximise the effectiveness of verbal and written communication within the staff team.

- Understand how to create partnerships with external professionals to benefit people with dementia.

- Recognise support needs of relatives and friends of people with dementia and know how to facilitate their positive involvement.

Person-centred dementia care relies on effective communication between all those who are involved. The starting point, as considered in Chapter 1, is the gathering and documenting of detailed information about the individual – a process that should involve everyone who works directly with people with dementia. Assessment can never be successful if it is seen only as a formal role, conducted by a senior person at the point of referral and subsequently on fixed occasions. In fact, assessment is a crucial aspect of the role of care staff and it is very important that leaders make this clear, that information discovered by staff is valued and that their efforts are praised.

CREATING EFFECTIVE CARE PLANS

It is only through gaining in-depth knowledge of individuals and how they relate to the world around them that we can avoid assumptions and make plans to meet individual needs. May, Edwards and Brooker (2009) explain the process of Enriched Care Planning, based on the understanding that each person's care and support needs arise from their own experience of dementia in terms of their life history, lifestyle and future wishes, personality, health, capacity and cognitive support needs and their life at the moment. The care plan is a key tool for communicating these needs with the team in order to ensure that the goals of care for each individual are identified and met.

Using the care plan as a tool for communication

Of course, what is most important is that staff know this information about individuals. Even in the absence of care plans, person-centred care can still take place if staff know people well and understand how to use their knowledge. But remembering in-depth information about a large number of people is not easy and, moreover, if this knowledge has not been recorded, person-centred care depends entirely consistency of personnel, which can never be guaranteed.

The purpose of a care plan is to guide care and interactions – information held on file means nothing if it is not used.

For example

Discovering that Charles is a keen Arsenal fan is relevant only if staff use this information to initiate conversations and remind him when matches are on TV.

Knowing that Gloria has full control of her continence but can't find the toilet is vital information because it enables care staff to provide essential guidance to help her maintain her dignity.

Sadly, rather than being appreciated as the vital guidelines they can be, all too often care plans are seen as time-consuming irritations, completed only because this is required by the regulatory body. So although written documentation of some kind will exist in every care service, it may do nothing to promote or enable person-centred care. At worst, some care plans are so generalised that if the client's name were to be removed, no-one could possibly guess whose plan it was. Some plans focus solely on problems and ignore strengths, are littered with negative terminology and sometimes even fundamental mistakes about, for example, an individual's family situation or their health needs. Often the very template on which care plans are composed leads away from person-centred practice – such as the commonly found heading 'Identified problem or need', which leads each section of the care plan off on a problem-centred focus.

Care plans can sometimes lead care astray through asserting mistaken assumptions, rooted in the kinds of negative beliefs described in Chapter 2. If the plan informs staff that Maud is 'often aggressive due to her dementia', for example, staff are diverted from the necessity of discovering the factors that distress her and will instead believe that her 'aggression' has no cause other than her illness. Moreover, 'aggression' is non-specific; it could mean anything from rude words to physical violence and could be the expression of a range of feelings, including fear, embarrassment and anger. The use of language will be further explored later in this chapter.

Even organisations that try to write person-centred care plans often end up with over-long documents that contain a dearth of usable information. A common shortfall identified by Walker and Manterfield (2010) is that the plan is too vague and lacks clarity. Phrases such as 'needs assistance with...', for example, offer no guidance to staff, who then have to make their own assumptions about the type and level of help that the person actually needs. 'Give support' is another ambiguous phrase frequently found in care plans, offering no information about how to support the individual. Instructions need to be specific if they are to be of any real use.

For example

'When Doris walks up and down looking anxious, walk with her for a while and then suggest going into her room to watch one of her DVDs – this usually helps her relax.'

'Put toothpaste on the toothbrush for Robert and hand it to him – then he is able to brush his own teeth.'

Auditing care plans

It is important that leaders seeking to develop person-centred dementia care practice devote some time to an audit of care plans – you may find it helpful to consider the questions in Table 5.1. Leaders also need to monitor the implementation of care plans and ensure that they are living documents, never at risk of gathering dust at the back of the filing cabinet.

Structuring care plans

Creating person-centred care plans is a challenge. Balanced against the importance of full and detailed guidelines on how to meet the person's needs, draw out their strengths, address their preferences and generally enhance their well-being, is the reality that if the plan is too long it will, quite simply, not be read. Some care services overcome this dilemma by creating some kind of summary sheet to go at the front of the care plan, containing key information about who the person is as an individual, and essential elements of their care needs. This can serve as a quick reference guide when urgently needed by a staff member who doesn't know the individual, but you must make sure that the whole care plan is read at a less pressurised time.

Table 5.1 A checklist for care plans

Care plans – a checklist

- Does each person's care plan identify the individual's strengths and abilities as well as their problems and difficulties?
- Do care plans address the needs of the whole person (not just their body)?
- Are care plans specific, giving details of what to do, when to do it, etc.?
- If the care service is full-time, does each care plan address the person's needs at night as well as throughout the day?
- Are care plans based on the person's wishes – preferences they've told staff about and/or things they've indicated non-verbally or through their behaviour?
- Is each care plan written in positive language, avoiding any negative labels or assumptions?
- Is each care plan unique? (Each person is unique, so their care plan should be different from everyone else's care plan.)
- Is each care plan regularly reviewed and dated? (Things can change quickly and it's important that any changes or new discoveries are quickly added to the care plan.)
- Are all the staff involved with each person familiar with what's in their care plan, and aware of when it's updated?
- Is each care plan practical and realistic – are staff members able to do what the care plan says they should do? (Do they have the time and skill to do it?)
- When individual staff members find out important information about an individual and how to meet their needs, does this information get incorporated into the care plan?
- Have the views of key people who know the individual (e.g. relatives) been taken into account in creating the care plan?
- Is each care plan seen as a valuable document in guiding care of the individual, or just an annoying bit of paperwork?

Walker and Manterfield (2010) stress the importance of separating assessment and planning information in order to declutter the plan of care. This also means that private information about the individual can be stored securely, while the 'hows' of care delivery can be kept in a place that is easily accessible to staff when they need to use it – for example, information about personal care can be kept in the individual's bedroom. One care home found that the most helpful place to put information about residents' clothing preferences and the assistance they needed with dressing was on a sheet taped to the inside of the person's wardrobe door.

In considering good practice regarding personal data, it is very important that the policy on confidentiality enables the sharing of information on a need-to-know basis. Home care staff must be fully briefed before visiting a new client; staff in care homes need access to any information that will help them support, interact with and care for individuals.

ENSURING EFFECTIVE DAY-TO-DAY COMMUNICATION BETWEEN STAFF

Good communication between staff is vital in any care service to ensure that care plans are up-to-date and everyone is fully aware of each individual's current needs.

Communicating verbally

It is important that staff know when and to whom different types of information should be communicated, and the need for clarity and accuracy when doing so. Misunderstandings can easily occur and both those conveying information and those receiving it must take responsibility for ensuring that it has been correctly understood. This is particularly important when anyone has English as a second language: those involved need to be prepared to double check that the peculiarities of the English language have not been misinterpreted. Misunderstandings can have serious consequences.

For example

A care home resident had just started on new medication for which drinking grapefruit juice was contraindicated. But when the team leader passed these instructions on to the resident's keyworker, 'grapefruit juice' was misunderstood as 'grape juice'. The wrong drink was withheld and the resident continued – until the mistake was discovered some time later – to drink what was now a potentially life-threatening morning glass of grapefruit juice.

Leaders should also be aware of the kinds of words and phrases that staff use when they are talking about people with dementia. This aspect of verbal communication is considered later in this chapter.

Communicating in writing

Putting things in writing helps to ensure that information has been clearly conveyed. In many care settings, care staff are responsible for providing a written record of the client's well-being and the care given – perhaps in the form of a communication book or daily log. These notes should indicate how successfully the person's needs (as outlined in their care plan) are being met and must include any information of concern, such as untoward incidents or signs of ill-health. These notes could become a legal document, used as evidence in a safeguarding investigation or at a coroner's court, for example, so it is essential that information is recorded clearly and accurately. On an everyday basis, daily written records and their verbal exchange – for example at a handover meeting in a care home – should ensure that information is not lost and that any changes are quickly addressed. Often, though, information recorded in these daily notes is very generalised: 'Slept and ate well, bowels opened, watching TV this afternoon' is a typical example. On closer scrutiny, such generalised comments may not even be accurate. 'Watching TV' often just means that the person was in the lounge and the television was on. The person might have been asleep, bored, upset or having an engaging chat with another resident – no-one will ever know.

Leading handover meetings

It is important to think about how full potential value can be derived from daily notes. It is most helpful if the limited time that is available for handing these notes over to colleagues is used to focus on new information that staff need to share and hear about.

For example

Jack has started on new medication that can cause nausea.

Eliza is very worried because her son has just been taken into hospital.

Hussein had a fall in the night and must be monitored to check for any adverse effects.

Rather than devoting any attention to mundane everyday occurrences, encourage specific exchanges about individuals, from which staff can learn. Information about someone opening their bowels or having a bath is not generally necessary to share, unless these activities are noteworthy for a particular person – such Cynthia, who has been constipated, or Max, who has previously refused to bathe. In these situations, more information should be drawn out to guide other staff towards the best approach.

For example

Has Cynthia's constipation been relieved because staff have managed to encourage her to eat more fruit and drink more fluids? How did they achieve this? What advice can they pass on?

Drawing out successes can help staff gain a deeper understanding of individual residents.

For example

The leader asks the care worker how he managed to encourage Max to have a bath and the care worker shares a vital piece of background information he discovered – that Max has been frightened of water since he was young and almost drowned in a river. As a result, Max is terrified by the prospect of getting into a full bath, but this morning, he seemed to feel fine about getting into an empty bath when the care worker promised that he would only fill it as far as Max wanted.

This is important information for all staff to know and utilise. A record should be kept of information that has been shared at the handover meeting, too, to help emphasise the responsibility of all present to use and act on it, and provide evidence of the information that staff have been given.

Time is generally short for handover meetings. They come at the end of a shift when staff are often anxious to leave work, so it is important to ensure that the meetings are time limited, focused and effectual. If the meeting becomes a forum where genuinely relevant and useful information is shared, it becomes a much more meaningful use of everyone's time and staff will understand the value of attending because it actually enables them to develop their practices and improve individuals' lives. In working to improve the quality of their handover meetings, leaders may need to think about structuring them differently or introducing particular discussions or activities to help staff get into new habits.

For example

Sue Heiser (to whom I am indebted for these thoughts on handover meetings), in her role as Service Manager for older people's homes in Camden, introduced an activity into handover meetings in one particular care home to encourage staff to engage more with residents and share ideas for how to do so: each staff member had to describe one interaction or activity they had done with a resident that day – a decent conversation, singing or dancing together or something that had not happened before.

Care that is truly centred on the person and responsive to their individual needs can only be achieved if everyone who works with that individual has an up-to-date understanding of how they are and what's been happening in their life. Things change frequently and person-centred care is responsive to these changes. The only way that a care plan can be current and relevant is if it is based on information provided by staff involved in their daily care.

Paying attention to language

The language we use when we communicate about people with dementia both reflects and influences attitudes and practices. Sometimes the language used about people with dementia is far from positive; you can often gain insight into the beliefs and priorities of staff through reading their entries in daily logs. 'Jane has been going round annoying other residents this morning', for example, reveals much about the staff member's attitude to and relationship with Jane. And if Jane is described as 'annoying', this may well impact on how others view her too, particularly staff who don't know Jane very well.

Then there are the labels that get applied to people whereby their diagnosis or behaviour becomes their primary feature – so Ruby is 'an Alzheimer's' and Tom is 'a wanderer'. The essence of their personhood is hidden from view. The term 'wandering' deserves a special mention, as it is an example of the unhelpful terminology that has evolved around dementia. In this instance, the very normal behaviour generally known as

> Listen to the words your staff use when talking about their work with people with dementia. What does this indicate about their attitudes?
>
> What about the language used in care plans and written notes?
>
> And what about the language you use? Does it reflect the approach that you are trying to promote?

'walking' has become pathologised – turned into a symptom. People with dementia walk for many reasons, just as we do – to go somewhere, to leave somewhere, to explore unfamiliar surroundings, to look for something, to get exercise, to manage pain, and so on. Sometimes, particularly if there's not much to do, any one of us, whether or not we have dementia, might 'wander' – i.e. walk with no particular purpose in mind. If a person with dementia is walking without purpose, then the word 'wandering' is accurate, but too often this word is used as a generalisation to describe a person with dementia walking for any reason at all. As such, it is misleading and distracts staff from the need to understand what it is that the person is seeking to do, where they want to go, and what this conveys about their needs. And, moreover, if 'wandering' is seen as a symptom or a meaningless behaviour, the focus will be on symptom or behaviour management, in the form of: 'Sit down Tom.'

The verbs that are used to describe the care process and approach are often very negative too. In some care homes, for example, staff will say that they have 'done' a resident – a shorthand way of saying that they have helped the person with their personal care, but a phrase that is also very suggestive of a task-focused, rather than person-focused, culture of care whereby the person themselves is seen as a job to do, akin to the bed that needs to be made and the floor that has to be swept. Many verbs used in the language of care imply passivity – 'I've fed Klara', for example, which conjures up a vivid image of disempowerment. A verb frequently found in care plans is 'allow' – as in 'Allow Fred to go to his room when he is tired.' Again this reveals something profound about the culture of care. If a person is 'allowed' to do something, then clearly someone else holds the power to decide whether this is permissible; at other times, actions the person wishes to take will inevitably be disallowed.

Leaders need to decide whether or not it will be helpful to challenge the language used by staff. There is certainly no point in telling staff what not to say without explaining why, and sometimes we need to choose our battles wisely: language may not be the most important one. Since words that are used are strongly influenced by the attitudes that lie underneath, changes in the culture of care will often be accompanied by gradual shifts in language occurring naturally. Rather than generalising about what 'they' like, for instance, as a person-centred approach becomes more instilled, staff will naturally speak more specifically about individuals. And staff who are actively working to enhance their clients' well-being are unlikely to refer to their clients as 'dementia sufferers'.

Whether or not leaders choose to take staff to task over the language they use, it is essential that you are mindful of the way you speak and write about people with dementia. Using positive, accurate and respectful language is an important aspect of your role modelling and helps to convey a consistent message about the attitudes with which staff are expected to provide care.

COMMUNICATING WITH EXTERNAL PROFESSIONALS

Accurate documentation and clear communication are never more important than when engaging with the wider multidisciplinary team involved in the care of the individual. In liaising with the district nurse, for example, or the general practitioner, it is essential that information about the person, their needs and their treatment, has been properly understood by all involved. As the dementia care leader it is important that you communicate clearly and assertively with the professional service regarding the person's specific needs, and any information about their preferences, beliefs, difficulties and strengths that the professional may need to work around or draw on.

In order to achieve maximum benefit for the person with dementia from the involvement of other professionals, the dementia care leader should work to develop partnerships, harnessing the strengths and knowledge of all parties involved.

For example

Doctors bring their medical knowledge and experience, but it is those who work closely with the person with dementia who have experience and detailed knowledge of the person as an individual. The needs and best interests of the person with dementia will best be served by combining both these areas of expertise.

To ensure that people with dementia benefit fully from the involvement of other professionals, dementia care leaders need to give careful thought, at the outset, to exactly why and whether the professional input is actually required and what specific needs it is hoped to address. Sometimes, for example, doctors are called to care homes because a resident's behaviour has become challenging. Now, the doctor might be the best person to consult, but only if the staff who are working closely with the individual have deduced that the change in behaviour is because the person is physically unwell or they are experiencing pain. This must be clearly communicated to the doctor – what physical symptoms the person has been experiencing, for example, or where in their body they are showing indications of pain. If, on the other hand, the doctor has been called to the care home because staff consider that 'challenging behaviour' is itself a problem that is likely to have a medical solution, the resident is unlikely to benefit from the visit. Either the doctor will recognise that there is no medical solution to offer, or they will feel obliged to prescribe medication – such as an antipsychotic – to try to stop the behaviour. Since this behaviour was communicating a message about something that was wrong, stopping the behaviour effectively means silencing the person's message without ever understanding it. The person's problem is unchanged – it is only their ability to try to make this known that has been altered. Dementia care leaders need to work closely with staff to help them develop their understanding of the wide range of messages that can be communicated through behaviour – this aspect of the leader's role is considered fully in Chapter 6.

It is always important to be aware of the roles that everyone involved must play in order to achieve the desired outcomes from professional input. The doctor prescribes a medicine, for example, but it is those in daily contact with the person who must be alert to its effects. The physiotherapist prescribes exercises, but care staff need to remind and assist the person to carry them out. At times, when involving external professionals, you may find that you have to tactfully share some of your own knowledge and experience of dementia. Unfortunately many professional education pathways fail to give students much understanding of dementia, and what they do know might be rooted in the medical model (as discussed in Chapter 2). Sometimes, you may need to advocate for the person with dementia, keeping a clear view of their capacity and best interests. You may need to request a medication review, for example, if you suspect that a person is not benefiting from certain medication they have been prescribed. At times, when dealing with rushed and harried visiting professionals, you may even need to explain the standards and procedures of the care service, to which they must also adhere. It contravenes policies of privacy and dignity, for example, if a district nurse changes somebody's dressings in the lounge of the care home – but they may need to be reminded of this. It will be even more helpful for the development of a mutually respectful relationship with the district nurse if staff help the resident to her bedroom prior to the nurse's visit.

In building effective partnerships with other professionals, it is important to gain their trust. The better your knowledge about the individuals receiving care from your service and the clearer your understanding about the goals of their care, the more likely the professional is to grow to trust your opinion and want to work cooperatively with you to achieve these goals.

COMMUNICATING WITH RELATIVES AND FRIENDS

Often, the key partnerships to be developed are with families and friends of people with dementia. Their knowledge regarding the person with dementia as an individual is vital to the process of person-centred care planning, but they may themselves need support. Staff often find that in order to enable the person with dementia to benefit from maintaining their closest relationships they have

How do you go about developing positive relationships with the relatives of your service users?

What support are you able to offer them?

What external sources of support and information are available in your area for relatives?

to be very sensitive and responsive in their contact with families. Relatives and other 'informal' carers of those with dementia often grapple with difficult feelings, and staff need to show empathy, not judgement, making it clear that they are taking the person's feelings seriously. Sometimes it may be appropriate to refer the relative to sources of outside help and advice, such as a dementia adviser or a carer support service.

While some relatives actively seek to inform themselves about dementia, others may have very little understanding and might benefit from information that you can provide. If you are able to offer group support, information or training sessions for relatives, there is the added advantage that people get to know others who are in a similar position. When giving information, it is important to be sensitive to the relative's feelings. For example, if a relative is feeling grief-stricken over their loved one's loss of abilities, it may not be helpful, at that point in time, to try to explain the signs of well-being that the person is showing. But for many relatives, it is uplifting if staff share positive information about things that the person has enjoyed or achieved.

For example

A care home had organised a swimming trip for a small group of residents with dementia. John's daughter doubted that he would be able to participate, but in the event, not only was he still able to swim, but also he took a leading role in encouraging another resident who was nervous. Even though John was unable to remember what he had eaten for breakfast, he remembered and talked about the swimming trip for many days afterwards. When this news was passed on to John's daughter, she was so pleased that there were tears in her eyes.

When relatives or friends are full-time or part-time carers, their lives may have become very stressful and exhausting. Practical support offered by a care agency or respite care service not only can help to address these needs, but also will often heighten feelings of guilt, shame and worry, and these feelings can get in the way of the relative being able to accept the help that is on offer. Some people have previously experienced care or respite services that have been of an inadequate standard and will understandably be worried about the competence of help that is now being offered. It is very important to try to adapt services to fit in with what is acceptable to the relative, recognising that it is only through the development of trust that the relative will be willing to let the care service gradually take on a larger role.

The troubling feelings mentioned earlier can sometimes impact on the relative's ability to help or interact with the person with dementia in the way the person needs. Sometimes, for example, relatives gradually withdraw from contact with the person with dementia, believing, perhaps, that since the person no longer recognises them, their visits are of no benefit. Some may believe that dementia has changed their relative so profoundly that the person they loved no longer exists; others might feel awkward when they do visit, not knowing how best to engage with someone who has lost many of their verbal communication skills. If at all possible, it is important to try to support the relative to overcome these feelings, encouraging them to maintain contact by helping them recognise how this benefits the person and perhaps by helping them find specific things to talk about or do when they visit – such as looking through a photo album. Of course family relationships are not always positive and for some, present relationships are shaped by a difficult history with the person who now has dementia. The relative may be striving to overcome very difficult feelings about the person and may need to speak about this – they may even need to be supported to withdraw from much or all of their contact with the person with dementia if neither party is benefiting.

Sometimes issues arise that challenge dementia care leaders to find ways of supporting relatives and family relationships while trying to manage the negative impact that is inadvertently being caused. For example, some relatives may take over and do everything for the person with dementia, thus unwittingly denying them the opportunity, and ultimately the ability, to do things for themselves. This kind of situation tends to arise because of the relative's fierce determination to demonstrate their love for the person with dementia through the care they give, so it would be heartless to blatantly point out how they are disempowering the person with dementia. Some relatives unintentionally cause stress for the person with dementia by insisting that they try to do things they can no longer do, arguing with them about things they've forgotten and telling them off for mistakes they've made. These interactions often come about because the relative is finding the person's loss of abilities so distressing that the only way they can cope emotionally is to deny that anything is wrong at all. In these kinds of situations, it can sometimes be helpful to gently offer advice, but it can be very difficult for relatives to accept that a new approach would be beneficial if it means confronting the possibility that their own might not have been for the best. It may be that the most appropriate strategy is simply to role model excellent care and communication and hope that the relative notices (or perhaps gently point out) any positive responses made by the person with dementia. If there are opportunities for the relative to participate in any kind of information or training session this can be very helpful too.

Some relatives, worried that the person with dementia is not receiving the best possible quality of care, can be perceived by care staff as highly critical. Others, particularly if they feel guilty about involving a care service or sanctioning the person's move into a care home, may seek to take control, from a distance, over the person's care. A daughter might try to insist, for example, that her mum has a bath every day – even though her mum much prefers to have a stand-up wash. It can be hard for care staff to develop good relationships with people's relatives if they are perceived to be unappreciative or critical, or in situations where there are tensions between the rights of the person with dementia and the approach or demands of the relative.

The dementia care leader can support staff by helping them understand the feelings that have led to the relative's behaviour and by suggesting proactive steps that could be taken to alter the relative's experience and enable them to develop trust in the care service. It is always important that the relative feels they are being listened to and respected, for example, and if the relative has criticisms to make about the care service, these must be taken seriously and responded to with openness and clarity. Sometimes it can be useful to offer practical help, advice or suggestions, explaining the values and goals underpinning the care approach, but it is also essential to validate the relative's input and role in the life of the person with dementia, to draw on their expertise about the person's life history, current needs and preferences and ensure that they feel recognised as the key people in the individual's life. Their input and advice when drawing up and reviewing care plans is vital.

So dementia care leaders have a key role in ensuring that excellent communication flows throughout the care service. From ensuring that everyone providing care has current and comprehensive information about individuals, to building bridges with others who impact on their lives, person-centred care cannot be a reality without effective communication.

Table 5.2 Chapter 5 key points

Key points	What leaders need to do
Care plans should be detailed plans of action that guide staff in meeting individuals' holistic needs	Write and regularly update care plans that are specific, comprehensive, positive and usable
Communication between staff should be clear and purposeful	Guide staff on what information is relevant and useful and needs to be passed on; ensure it is understood by all who need to know it
Language used about people with dementia can both indicate and influence attitudes	Use positive, non-labelling and respectful language at all times when talking or writing about people with dementia
Leaders can help the involvement of external professionals bring positive results for people with dementia	Ensure that referrals are appropriate; communicate clearly and assertively regarding the person as an individual and their specific needs
Leaders should aim to develop partnerships with the relatives and friends of people with dementia	Provide emotional support, value their knowledge, offer guidance and information if necessary and facilitate their involvement as active partners in the process of care

Chapter 6

Working Together to Respond to Feelings and Needs

By the end of this chapter, you will:

- Have considered the importance of empathising with staff who are feeling challenged by behaviour.
- Understand some of the feelings and needs that can lie behind behaviour, and help staff empathise.
- Have some methods to help with problem-solving in teams.
- Know how to support staff to respond constructively to behaviour.
- Understand what is involved in person-centred risk assessment and management.

One of the key indicators of a person-centred dementia care service is its ability to understand and constructively respond to people's feelings. A dementia care leader who is making an effort to prioritise and value communication knows that people communicate their feelings in a myriad of ways. When verbal abilities are compromised, people do not stop communicating but they use any means they can to convey their meaning, through actions, sounds, expressed emotions and any language that remains.

Bryden (2005, p.128) gives the example: 'People make you do things that you don't want to do, and you have no word for "No, thank you." So all you can do is push them out of the way because they want to shower or dress you, or give you food you don't like.' But messages communicated in this way can easily be misconstrued or dismissed as 'challenging behaviours', assumed to be symptoms of dementia, in need of being controlled or managed. As we have seen in Chapter 4, this mistaken assumption blocks the learning cycle and poses a significant barrier to person-centred care. If we seek to 'manage' behaviour rather than understand its meaning, we are likely to miss out on vital information the person with dementia is trying to give us about their feelings and needs.

UNDERSTANDING BEHAVIOUR THAT CHALLENGES STAFF
Empathising with staff

Person-centred dementia care leaders must search for a balance whereby they emphasise the importance of recognising these feelings and needs, and simultaneously empathise with staff who are facing behaviours they find difficult, stressful or even threatening. Many staff working in dementia care settings regularly feel challenged by the way people with dementia express themselves. The experience of living with dementia and having to receive help from others often provokes strong feelings such as frustration, distress and anxiety, and to be faced with people expressing such feelings – and doing so in a context where, through dementia, they have probably lost some of their inhibitions – can indeed be difficult. Staff might find themselves being shouted or sworn at, being racially abused or even physically hurt. Leaders must take such experiences seriously – to neglect the reality of staff in these kinds of situations and leave them feeling unsupported would defeat the possibility that staff could ever develop the ability and willingness to provide emotional support to people with dementia. This is important even when the staff member has inadvertently provoked the challenging behaviour that has distressed them.

So, as I discussed in Chapter 3, leaders need to give time and attention to staff and be prepared to listen with empathy and without judgement. There may also be action that you need to take to make it clear that you are serious about supporting staff – for

> What behaviours do your staff find challenging?
>
> What messages do you think are being communicated through these behaviours?

example speaking to the client who has been racially abusive and explaining that this is not acceptable. It may be unlikely that the client will remember the conversation or be able to modify their behaviour accordingly, but it is important to demonstrate to staff that you are taking the matter seriously. Your conversation with the client might also provide an opportunity for you to hear directly from them, if they are able to remember, about what it was that upset them. It is also very helpful to get directly involved and work alongside the staff member in the situation that provoked the challenging reaction. This is useful both in terms of helping staff feel supported and also giving you a clearer understanding of what triggers the client's behaviour and what they are communicating through it. With this enhanced understanding you may be able to help the staff member find out how to avoid similar stresses in the future.

Helping staff empathise with people with dementia

Something important to bear in mind is that while the ongoing losses involved in living with dementia are in themselves hard to cope with, further stresses are posed by the misunderstandings and mistakes that arise because of these losses.

For example

People often have difficulty negotiating their environment, resulting, for example, in someone going into another person's bedroom instead of their own, or urinating in a lift, believing it to be a toilet.

People can easily misinterpret a situation, believing their care worker to be a stranger, thinking that clothes taken to the laundry have been stolen, or mistaking a personal care intervention as a sexual advance. It is then likely that people will act on such beliefs by fighting the stranger off, accusing the thief, or responding to their seducer.

Such reactions, so often misinterpreted as examples of personality change, are in fact completely understandable when viewed within the context of the person's difficulties and their perception of their situation. Bryden says, 'For people with dementia our behaviour is normal, considering what is happening inside our heads. Try to enter our distorted reality, because if you make us fit in with your reality, it will cause us extra stress' (Bryden 2005, p.147). The 'distorted reality' can also lead people with dementia to express their needs in ways that relate to their past rather than their present life: a need for comfort might be expressed through someone calling for their mother; a need to be occupied might lead someone out of their front door at 7 a.m., believing they are going to work.

Such situations can easily make dementia care a battleground if staff are not mindful of their own communication and behaviour and alert to the support that people need. Explanations might need to be frequently repeated; introductions might need to take place at the beginning of every interaction. A high degree of empathy is required in order to try, as Bryden (2005) instructs us, to enter the reality of the person with dementia. As mentioned earlier, it is vital for you to role model this process in your interactions with staff – by showing that you can see things from the staff member's perspective. The methods for guiding reflective practice, discussed in Chapter 4, will also be key to moving forward. This would involve asking the staff member to think about what the client's viewpoint and beliefs might be and how they think the person is feeling.

For example

'What might Mavis be communicating through her behaviour?'

'Why do you think Patrick is asking for his mother? What might he need from her?'

Using the insights gained from considering questions such as these, staff can begin to think creatively about ways of addressing people's underlying needs and making situations less stressful for people with dementia.

Problem-solving in teams

When there is a problem, it is generally useful to involve staff in a discussion about it. One of the first steps may be to analyse exactly why it is a problem. Sometimes, for example, a person's behaviour is causing concern simply because their standards or preferences are different to those of the staff member involved. It might be hard, for instance, for a home care worker who is herself very neat and tidy to accept the messy home environment in which her client feels comfortable; another staff member may feel very uncomfortable about his client's sexual preferences and see this issue as a problem. But unless the client's choices pose an unreasonable health or safety risk and the person lacks the mental capacity to make their own decision about this, it would not be appropriate to seek to alter the person's behaviour or their environment. What needs to change in both these situations is the staff member's acceptance that everyone has the right to their own standards. Leaders may find that this requires a lot of talking and time, particularly if the staff member has deep-seated beliefs on the issue of concern.

Team discussion can also be particularly helpful in situations where the 'problem' associated with a person's behaviour is not a problem for the person themselves, but for staff or other people.

For example

Antonio, who used to be an odd-job man, frequently went into other residents' bedrooms to see if anything needed fixing. He was expressing his well-being, but other residents were upset. Through discussing ways of enabling Antonio to constructively use his sense of purpose and desire to be helpful, staff came up with various ideas, including the handyman regularly asking for his assistance with straightforward maintenance jobs.

It may be quite straightforward to understand why somebody has behaved in a particular way. Clearly Antonio's previous job was a key contributory factor, for instance. Often, with observational skills and a good knowledge of the person and the situation, we will be able to pinpoint the reasons for a person's behaviour.

For example

We can see from Bernard's body language – and perhaps he is even able to tell us – that he is walking up and down because he is in pain.

We can understand that Edna lashed out because a care worker unthinkingly approached her from behind and startled her.

Sometimes it is not easy to interpret why the person with dementia has behaved as they have. Gaining an understanding of the more complex causes of challenging behaviour is a process that is often most successfully undertaken in a group. More heads are better than one, as long as the leader can prompt constructive thinking.

Are there any current situations where the reasons for a person's behaviour are not apparent?

Try 'creative brainstorming' with your team...how many possible reasons can be identified through this?

'Creative brainstorming', as suggested by Stokes (2000), is a useful method for doing this. This involves working together to generate as many explanations for a person's behaviour as can be found, including those that seem improbable, and then investigating any that are even remotely possible. Stokes gives an example of the 94 possible reasons identified by a staff team for a particular resident's refusal to get out of bed (Stokes 2000, pp.137–140), and explains how any of these that were remotely possible were investigated, with the actual reasons eventually being pinpointed and resolved.

Stokes (2000) also emphasises the importance of considering all the factors that might individually, or in conjunction with others, trigger an individual's behaviour – from health problems to care practices, from the physical surroundings to the person's life history. As we considered in Chapter 1, a wide range of factors can cause problems for people with dementia. Working together to consider the questions in Table 6.1 can help a team to consider the range of reasons that could be contributing to an individual's behaviour and avoid making assumptions.

Table 6.1 Identifing and addressing needs communicated through behaviour

1. Could the person's behaviour result directly from a symptom of their dementia? *(e.g. the person has perceptual problems and this causes them to mistake a chair for a toilet)*	If so, what extra help does the person need to compensate for their symptoms?
2. In addition to their dementia, does the person have any physical/sensory problems that could influence their behaviour? *(e.g. hearing impairment that means the person can't hear explanations given, being in pain, poor mobility that makes the person feel trapped, etc.)*	If so, how could these be better addressed?
3. Is there anything that staff do that seems to trigger the person's behaviour? *(e.g. approaching the person from behind, speaking loudly, not giving the person sufficient time to understand what's happening, giving too much help, etc.)*	If so, how could this be changed?
4. Is there anything in the person's social world that might trigger their behaviour? *(e.g. a personality clash with another client or a neighbour, a regular visitor being on holiday, etc.)*	If so, how could this be addressed?
5. Is there anything in the environment that you think might influence the person's behaviour? *(e.g. noisy environment, confusing layout, lots of people around, warm/cold environment, sitting in a particular place, etc.)*	If so, how could this be changed?
6. Is there anything you know about the person's life history that could be triggering the person's behaviour? *(e.g. preferring to be alone rather than with others, having been abused as a child, having been the victim of a crime, a previous job or routine that involved an aspect of the behaviour, etc.)*	If so, how could you use your understanding of this to adapt your communication and/or their plan of care?
7. What messages about their FEELINGS and NEEDS do you think the person is communicating through their behaviour? *(These messages could be negative (e.g. about feelings of fear) or positive (e.g. the person could be communicating that they like to feel useful))*	What immediate responses might help? What long-term responses might help to meet the person's needs and prevent the difficult feelings from reoccurring?

RESPONDING TO PROBLEMS

Addressing the factors that have triggered behaviour

Pinpointing the reasons for a person's behaviour does not always offer an instant solution but it may well suggest a course of action. Clearly Bernard needs to see a doctor about his pain, and staff must avoid approaching Edna from behind. In situations where someone's challenging behaviour seems to have been triggered by the approach of a particular staff member, it is important to be aware that this is very likely to have happened inadvertently. Leaders must steer well away from blaming anyone for causing a person with dementia to react in a challenging way. Humiliating or chastising the staff member for this is unlikely to help them learn from their mistake and will, moreover, make them and other staff less likely to openly discuss challenging situations again. Leaders must maintain a supportive approach, gently helping staff to recognise the unintended effect of their actions within the context of encouraging them to find an alternative approach.

To understand the part that the environment might play in affecting behaviour, it is important to understand the person's symptoms and how these are likely to alter their relationship with their surroundings.

For example

With impaired short-term memory and orientation, how will the person be able to find their way around? Is there any way of knowing which bedroom is theirs, or where the toilet is?

With impaired perceptual abilities, how can the person make sense of their environment? Are there patterns in the carpet that could be seen as something growing out of the floor, or shadows that might look like holes? Are there small flowers on the duvet cover that might be mistaken for insects?

With a decreased ability to perceive colour contrasts and depth, is it evident where the floor ends and the toilet begins?

If someone is not able to recognise their own reflection, will they be likely to know that the person they see in the bathroom is not another resident, but themselves?

If something about the environment has triggered a person's challenging behaviour, it is important to be flexible and creative in considering how changes could be made. It may be that there is something immediately achievable that could resolve the problem – putting a clear sign on the person's bedroom door, for example, or changing the bedcover that is causing distress. The mirror could be removed or covered; a brighter bulb could be fitted. Some aspects of the environment are not easily changed – a long corridor, for example, that increases disorientation – but there are various steps that can be taken to make this more manageable for people with dementia, such as introducing seating areas along the way and putting up attention-grabbing pictures to serve both as landmarks and items of interest.

When the main trigger to a person's challenging behaviour seems to be an aspect of their own life history, this cannot be changed, but with an understanding of the person's past, it is often possible to find ways of avoiding the trigger and/or addressing the person's needs.

For example

Nancy became highly agitated when in the company of anyone wearing black clothing, because she was reminded of the long period of mourning she had gone through when a number of her family members died in a fire. It was not difficult for staff to dress differently when visiting her.

Bill, because he had been a security guard, was not willing to go to bed at night until he had checked that all windows and doors were locked. Staff incorporated this into his nightly routine.

Responding to problems that can't be 'fixed'

Thus sometimes, having pinpointed the reasons for a person's behaviour, there is an immediate response that is likely to help. But some problems do not have solutions. Let us consider Phillip, for example, who spends his day in a state of restless anxiety because he is aware of his progressive loss of abilities and finds this distressing and frightening. There is no straightforward way of altering the reality of Phillip's situation: it is understandable that with his level of insight, dementia is emotionally very difficult to deal with.

It is also often emotionally difficult for staff when there isn't a solution to the person's problems. If they can't fix what's wrong, they may feel that they can't help at all. However, you need to support staff to recognise how important it is for them to 'be there' for Phillip, paying close attention, offering non-judgemental acceptance and showing that they care. His problems are still there, but for Phillip, being able to express his feelings to someone who listens and tries to understand may bring a sense of relief and the comfort of knowing he is not alone. As discussed in Chapter 3, leaders need to offer emotional support to staff to enable them to provide and maintain this kind of empathy. Furthermore, you need to give practical consideration to how it can be made possible for them to do this. It may be helpful to allocate specific responsibilities around an individual's emotional support needs to one or two staff members, who will try to develop closer relationships with the person. This can be enabled by organising the daily schedule so that these staff have some time available each day to give the person focused one-to-one attention.

It is also important that the wider team is aware of the feelings and needs of someone who is very troubled. A consistent approach, implemented by all staff, is necessary. If all staff regularly praise Phillip's achievements and draw out his strengths, there is the highest possibility that, over time, Phillip's anxiety will ease.

WORKING WITH RISK

Some of the most difficult situations to respond to are when a person's behaviour poses a risk to their own or someone else's health or safety. Here, some different challenges come into play. Clearly dementia care leaders have a responsibility towards the safety of their clients but it is never possible to protect a person from every eventuality, nor would it be in their best interests to do so. Risk is a part of life and we cannot eliminate risk for people with dementia, but our society has a tendency towards over-protecting older people in general, and people with dementia in particular. Too often, the focus of risk management in dementia care is on how to prevent people from engaging in activities that pose a risk of harm. Stopping people from doing the things they want to do often results in quality of life deteriorating; this negative impact of not taking the risk has been termed by Clarke *et al.* (2011, p.61) as 'silent harm'. The real challenge is to find ways of managing the risks so that the person is enabled to live in a way that matches their preferences and needs as closely as possible.

The process of risk management must take place within the framework of legislation that protects people's rights – for example in England and Wales, the Mental Capacity Act 2005, which upholds a person's rights to make their own decisions where they have the capacity to do so, and the Mental Health Act 2007, which introduced safeguards to protect people from being inappropriately deprived of their liberty. Too often, people with dementia fall prey to assumptions of incapacity made by everyone from family members to social care professionals. Dementia care leaders may need to recognise and present evidence that an individual is able to make a particular decision. The Mental Capacity Act 2005 also ensures that if a person lacks capacity to make a particular decision, any decision made on their behalf must be made in their best interests and the least restrictive of their basic rights and freedoms. Such decision-making is an important responsibility for dementia care leaders. The consideration of a person's 'best interests' needs to take into account the psychological, social and cultural impact of decisions – monitoring the person's well-being (a process described in Chapter 1) can be helpful in assessing this.

Assessing individual risk

Leaders need to be thoughtful and well informed when assessing risk and planning strategies for managing it. It is particularly important to gather specific information about the individual's difficulties which impact on the level and type of risk involved in an activity, and their abilities that serve as resources in the risky situation (Littlechild and Blakeney 1996). Equally importantly, we need to consider the context within which the activity is taking place.

For example

Esther lives in a care home and wishes to go out on a daily basis to the local shops. The fact that Esther has dementia should not, in itself, be seen as a reason to prevent Esther from going out. But concerns have arisen because on two occasions Esther has been unable to find her way home. On the other hand, she has good mobility and retains all her abilities related to crossing roads. Her verbal communication skills are intact and she is alert and self-aware. In terms of the context, Esther lives in a care home in a fairly quiet residential area; there is only one group of shops nearby, all adjacent.

It has been suggested (Nuffield Council on Bioethics 2009) that the process of risk assessment can be usefully seen as a process of weighing up 'harms' against 'benefits' (see Figure 6.1). Aspects of the risk that could potentially weigh down the 'harms' involve both the severity and the likelihood of negative outcomes occurring. With detailed knowledge of Esther's difficulties and abilities, the dementia care leader can assess that the likelihood of any severe harm (such as Esther getting hit by a car) is no greater than for anyone without dementia. The risk of her getting lost is more substantial, but is unlikely to lead to injury, particularly since her alertness and her communication abilities enable her to recognise when she is lost, and to ask for directions. Furthermore, if the likelihood of Esther getting lost is analysed, we notice that this has happened only twice before. It is important to check daily records from these occasions; there may be specific reasons to be found, such as Esther being in the early stages of an infection and more confused as a result. If this is the case, then the risk of this happening again, as long as Esther is well, is negligible. The environmental context of the quiet residential location of the care home further decreases the likelihood of Esther coming to harm even if she does get lost.

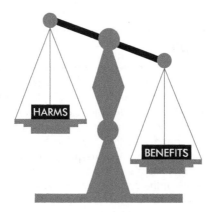

Figure 6.1: Harms vs. benefits

It can be seen, then, that in Esther's case the 'harms' side of the balance is not heavy, and if we consider the benefits that counterbalance it – for instance her sense of independence, her self-confidence, being occupied in doing something purposeful, feeling a part of her community and gaining physical exercise – then going out to the shops is clearly in Esther's best interests.

In situations where the likelihood or severity of harm outweighs the benefits that could be derived from taking the risk, it is essential to ensure that the person's needs are addressed in alternative ways. If Esther were to lose the abilities that have enabled her to go out to the shops on her own, the care home would need to identify alternative purposeful activities to address her needs for confidence, independence, socialisation and exercise.

> Consider a current situation where there are concerns that a person is at risk...
>
> What are the 'harms' that could occur?
>
> How likely are these?
>
> What benefits does the person derive from the behaviour that puts them at risk?

Managing risk

But while the future should be kept in mind, it is important that risk management plans are grounded in the present, acknowledging the person's current level of abilities. The risk assessment of Esther's daily walks has determined that for the time being it is in her best interests to continue, so what is crucial is that a clear plan is developed that identifies how Esther will be supported to do this and to remain as safe as possible.

For example

Staff can log the time of Esther's departure and note what she is wearing (just in case there is a need to search for her later on). They can offer Esther the care home's name and address on a card to keep in her pocket or handbag, and swap phone numbers with the local shopkeepers.

Since people's abilities are likely to change, it is of course critical that there are strategies to quickly pick up on these changes so that any necessary measures to manage increases in risk can be swiftly put in place. The risk management plan therefore needs to include ways of checking its own effectiveness and continued applicability. Frequent monitoring of the person's abilities and regular reviews of the plan are essential; it will be vital, for example, to pick up on any evidence that Esther is beginning to lose her sense of road safety and put a new plan in place.

A risk management plan also needs to consider ways in which the environment might need to be adapted to prevent unnecessary risks and enable people to be as independent as possible.

For example

When seeking to manage the risks involved in cooking, it will be important to ensure that all the equipment the person needs is familiar in design and is easy to find – glass-fronted cupboard doors can be helpful.

If a person is at risk of falling it is particularly important that floor coverings are plain, lighting is good and there is effective use of colour and signage to help the person find their way without stress.

In group care settings, there are sometimes important discussions to be had about how the environment can best suit the needs of all the clients. A locked front door, for instance, might cause frustration for able clients such as Esther, but might be necessary in order to ensure the safety of clients who lack the ability to go out safely on their own. It is always helpful to consider whether the use of assistive technology could help to resolve the situation – perhaps a device linked to the handle of the front door could alert staff to a client's desire to leave the building so that they can intervene as appropriate.

Assistive technology can play a key role in the management of risk and the enablement of people with dementia, not only by alerting staff to the fact that a person may need some assistance – such as the device on the front door or a sensor that tells staff when a person has got out of bed – but also in helping people live more independently. Devices can be used to compensate for memory deficits, for example, such as a pill dispenser that reminds the person when to take their medication or a bath plug that automatically releases excess water if the taps have been left running. It is useful for dementia care leaders to inform themselves about the range of assistive technology devices that are available, for example by browsing the AT dementia website (www.atdementia.org.uk).

Working collaboratively

Supporting individuals to take reasonable risks is most likely to succeed when the decision-making process has involved all those who have an interest in the person's care, including their family, who may need support in understanding that it is neither possible nor desirable to eliminate risk altogether. You may be the one who has to advocate for individuals' rights to take reasonable risks, but it is important that decisions are made collaboratively and are recorded. Team members need to understand the reasons for decisions that are made, and this is most likely to happen when they have been able to contribute their views, air their feelings and hear the opinions of others. Some people are naturally more risk averse than others. Staff who have had a previous experience of a person with dementia coming to harm in a similar situation may need help to recognise ways in which the current situation is different. Esther is not the same as any other client; her exact combination of abilities and difficulties is unique, as are her wishes, her personality and her situation.

In working with a team to make plans for managing the challenges posed by risk, staff may need to be assured that they will not be blamed should there be a negative outcome, as long as they have fulfilled their responsibilities. However, the buck does have to stop somewhere, and dementia care leaders who hold senior management positions will be the people who are likely to be called to account if things go wrong. While this is not a welcome prospect, as long as a full risk assessment has been undertaken and documented and a detailed plan has been created to explain how the risk will be managed, the leader should have nothing to fear. It is appropriate, in order to safeguard the rights of vulnerable people, that questions should be asked and decisions scrutinised. Indeed, it is precisely to safeguard the rights of these same individuals that we are seeking to enable them rather than to restrict them unnecessarily and deny their quality of life. It is quite right that leaders should be accountable: what is unfortunate is that there is not generally a similar level of enquiry when a person with dementia is damaged by the silent harms inflicted by leaders who opt for safety at any price.

CONCLUSION

In general, the amount of 'challenging behaviour' from people with dementia is strongly influenced by the style of care and the level of empathic awareness. When staff understand the realities of living with dementia, they tend to be more accepting and supportive of people expressing feelings, and it is less likely that these feelings will escalate and cause problems. And when staff are able to 'reflect in action' and adjust their interactions with the person with dementia according to the individual's responses, there will be less provocation of defensive reactions, higher self-esteem and lower levels of distress and frustration. A clear understanding of the goals for dementia care will also make a big difference to how staff view people's behaviour. For example, an understanding that a person with dementia who is being assertive about their own preferences and choices is clearly displaying a sense of well-being means that 'non-cooperation' is not seen as a problem, but rather staff are glad that the person is not meekly accepting the choices that others may want to make for them.

For dementia care leaders seeking to find the best way of guiding a staff team towards a better approach to challenging situations, it is important to recognise that every aspect of dementia care leadership explored earlier in this book will have a bearing on this – from ensuring that staff understand the goals of dementia care, to creating care plans that highlight abilities and document individual preferences. Sometimes it is through tackling challenges together with staff that leaders really have an opportunity to influence attitudes and approaches. The 'problem' can be the catalyst that prompts a deeper level of insight or that steers a team towards more cooperative work practices.

Table 6.2 Chapter 6 key points

Key points	What leaders need to do
The experience of living with dementia often provokes strong feelings which may be expressed in ways that staff find challenging	Empathise with staff and support them to empathise with people with dementia
A variety of factors may trigger an individual to behave in a way that staff find challenging	Lead a team-focused problem-solving approach and consider changes – e.g. to the environment – that might be helpful
Risk is a part of life and we need to focus on enablement rather than restriction	Gather specific information and weigh up the balance of harms and benefits to find a course of action that promotes the person's best interests
People with dementia should be supported to be as safe as possible while taking risks that benefit them	Collaboratively develop a plan that may include compensatory strategies, environmental modifications and assistive technology

Conclusion
Moving Forward

The more that is written and evidenced about good practice in dementia care, the more imperative it becomes that we are equipped to lead this good practice. I have earlier argued that person-centred dementia care does not exist, in any consistent form, without person-centred dementia care leadership. The issues are too complex, the challenges too multifarious. Good training for person-centred care is important, but alongside this is the necessity of guidance, support and inspiration from within the workplace. Person-centred care is all about people – not only those with dementia, but also those who are caring for them – and dementia care leaders must take to heart the challenge of enabling all of these individuals to develop their full potential.

FACING THE CHALLENGE OF LEADERSHIP

The role of the person-centred dementia care leader involves working to hold onto and address many different needs, feelings and views, and simultaneously to influence them. Your role is multifaceted and demanding. Many of the challenges you face are intense and complex and many of the needs for which you are responsible are profound. And you are probably doing this within a context where resources are insufficient and the claims on your time are many and varied.

Some leaders describe themselves as jugglers – keeping many balls in the air and catching them before they fall. Others have likened their role to that of a gardener, who sows, nurtures and tends; who battles against weeds and pests. Clearly you need tenacity and commitment in order to meet the challenge and reap the rewards. And it is essential, as a leader, that you hold firmly onto hope.

It is also very important that you find sources of support for yourself, both from within your organisation and externally. It can help both to sustain you and to prompt creative thinking if you can meet and share ideas with leaders from other services – for example within the context of care forums, workforce development collaboratives, or dementia focus groups, if anything like these exist in your area. Seeking out training opportunities and going to conferences can also be useful ways of finding like-minded people who are grappling with some of the same challenges. And – essentially – within your care service itself, through developing a culture of open communication and reflective practice, you can draw out the best ideas and efforts of your staff, thereby creating allies to strengthen your efforts and fuel your momentum.

ACTION PLANNING

I have earlier described the process of creating a person-centred dementia care service as a journey. It is essential not only to keep focused on the destination, but also to plan the route. If your destination were the summit of a mountain, you would need landmarks and way posts – places you could aim for on the long walk up and where you could stop, take breath and admire the view. You'd need to be realistic about how long it would be likely to take to reach the top, given the height of the mountain and your own fitness and strength, and you'd need to work out how far you could go at a time. I could extend the metaphor further and stress the importance of taking your waterproofs and sandwiches...but I'm sure you get the point!

If your vision for the future of your care service is the mountain top, you need to plan the more immediate objectives to aim for and make sure they are 'SMART' – Specific, Measurable, Attainable, Relevant and Time-bound (Meyer 2003). You could aim, for example, that within the next year all your staff will have a comprehensive understanding of the goals of person-centred care. Having pinpointed the objective, you will need to identify the steps that have to be taken to achieve it. The first step might be sourcing and costing an appropriate training course, and the second might be to write this cost into your budget, or to negotiate with whoever holds the purse strings. Subsequent steps will need to address how you will ensure that all staff attend the course, how you will keep alive the lessons learnt, how you will prompt new learning through reflective practice, what targets you will set for each individual to put what they have learnt into action, how you will monitor this, how you will involve staff in the process of monitoring, and so on.

The 'attainable' aspect of your objectives is important. Your targets should be demanding, but if they are too ambitious you are unlikely to reach them, which would be disheartening for you and your allies and could sap motivation. If, taking a pragmatic overview of the current state of attitudes and care in your organisation, your ultimate vision is so distant as to feel virtually unreachable, you don't need to alter your long-range aspirations, but your current working objectives might need to be realistically minimalist. It is much more beneficial to achieve and highlight small successes than to aim too high and render anything that has been attained along the way as a disappointment. Small wins will spur staff on to do more and achieve bigger things.

In any dementia care service, it is the experience of individual people with dementia that must be at the heart of your efforts. The underlying reason for all the objectives you set is to improve life for individuals, and there is no better place than this to start. Focus on one person with dementia; identify one area of the person's well-being that you think could be improved. Involve staff in discussing strategies for doing so; support them in implementing these strategies.

And when you succeed in improving the well-being of one person with dementia, know that you have achieved something that is profoundly important. It is transformational for the person's quality of life; inspirational for staff morale and learning. And it has brought you one hugely significant step closer to the achievement of your vision.

> Early one morning a man went for a walk on the beach. It was a wide, sandy beach that stretched for miles and even though it was early, the sun was already beating down. But the man noticed that dotted along the sand, as far as the eye could see, were thousands upon thousands of starfish that had been washed up onto the beach overnight. The starfish were dying as they lay in the burning rays of the morning sun.
>
> Then the man noticed a young boy ahead of him on the beach. As he watched, the boy bent down, picked up a starfish and threw it into the sea. Then he did the same with another, and another.
>
> As the man drew close to the boy, he said, 'Young man, why are you doing this? Look along the beach – see how many starfish there are! You can't possibly make a difference!'
>
> For a moment, the boy looked sad. But then he bent down, picked up another starfish and threw it as far as he could into the sea. 'Well, I made a difference to that one,' he said.

A retelling of *The Star Thrower* by Loren C. Eiseley (1978)

References

Adams, T. (2008) 'Nursing People with Dementia and their Family Members.' In T. Adams (ed.) *Dementia Care Nursing*. London: Macmillan.

Ajzen, I. and Fishbein, M. (2005) 'The Influence of Attitudes on Behaviour.' In D. Albarracín, B.T. Johnson and M.P. Zanna (eds) The *Handbook of Attitudes*. Mahwah, NJ: Lawrence Erlbaum.

Alzheimer's Disease International (2009) *World Alzheimer Report*. Chicago, IL: International Federation of Alzheimer's Disease and Related Disorders Societies. Available at www.alz.co.uk/research/files/World AlzheimerReport.pdf, accessed on 27 March 2012.

Alzheimer's Society (2007) *Home from Home: Quality of Care for People with Dementia Living in Care Homes*. London: Alzheimer's Society.

Asch, S.E. (1951) 'Effects of Group Pressure upon the Modification and Distortion of Judgment.' In H. Guetzkow (ed.) *Groups, Leadership and Men*. Pittsburgh, PA: Carnegie Press.

AT Dementia (n.d.) *Information on Assistive Technology for People with Dementia*. Leicester: Trent Dementia Services Development Centre. Available at www.atdementia.org.uk/default.asp, accessed on 27 March 2012.

Ballard, C. and Aarsland, D. (2009) 'Person-centred care and care mapping in dementia.' *The Lancet – Neurology 8*, 4, 302–303.

BBC News (2008) *Dementia Patients' 'Right-to-Die'*. London: BBC. Available at http://news.bbc.co.uk/1/hi/health/7625816.stm, accessed on 26 March 2012.

Beckford, M. (2008) 'Baroness Warnock: Dementia sufferers may have a "duty to die".' *The Telegraph*. Available at www.telegraph.co.uk/news/ uknews/2983652/Baroness-Warnock-Dementia-sufferers-may-have-a-duty-to-die.html, accessed on 26 March 2012.

Bonaparte, Napolean. In P. Holden (1998) *The Excellent Manager's Companion*. Hampshire: Gowen Publishing Ltd.

Brooker, D. (2007) *Person-Centred Dementia Care: Making Services Better*. London: Jessica Kingsley Publishers.

Brooker, D. and Surr, C. (2005) *Dementia Care Mapping: Principles and Practice*. Bradford: Bradford Dementia Group.

Brooker, D., Foster, N., Banner, A., Payne, M. and Jackson, L. (1998) 'The efficacy of Dementia Care Mapping as an audit tool: Report of a 3-year British NHS evaluation.' *Aging and Mental Health 2*, 1, 60–70.

Bryden, C. (2005) *Dancing with Dementia*. London: Jessica Kingsley Publishers.

Chalfont, G. (2008) *Design for Nature in Dementia Care*. London: Jessica Kingsley Publishers.

Chenoweth, L., King, M.T., Jeon, Y.H., Brodaty, H., Stein-Parbury, J., Haas, M., *et al.* (2009) 'Caring for Aged Dementia Care Resident Study (CADRES) of person-centred dementia care, dementia-care mapping, and usual care in dementia: A cluster-randomised trial.' *The Lancet – Neurology 8*, 4, 317–325.

Christian, D. (1997) 'Protecting her personal source of love.' *Journal of Dementia Care 5*, 4, 24–25.

Clarke, C.L., Wilkinson, H., Keady, J. and Gibb, C. (2011) *Risk Assessment and Management for Living Well with Dementia*. London: Jessica Kingsley Publishers.

Department of Health (2009) *Living Well with Dementia: A National Dementia Strategy*. London: Department of Health.

Eisley, L.C. (1978) *The Star Thrower*. New York: Times Books (Random House).

Festinger, L. (1957) *A Theory of Cognitive Dissonance*. Stanford, CA: Stanford University Press.

Fossey, J. and James, I. (2008) *Evidence-based Approaches for Improving Dementia Care in Care Homes*. London: Alzheimer's Society.

Iuppa, N.V. (1986) *Management by Guilt and Other Uncensored Tactics*. New York: Fawcett Crest.

Jolley, D. (2005) 'Why Do People with Dementia Become Disabled?' In M. Marshall (ed.) *Perspectives on Rehabilitation and Dementia*. London: Jessica Kingsley Publishers.

King's Fund (1986) *Living Well into Old Age: Applying Principles of Good Practice to Services for People with Dementia*. London: King's Fund.

Kitwood, T. (1993) 'Person and process in dementia.' *International Journal of Geriatric Psychiatry 8*, 7, 541–545.

Kitwood, T. (1995) 'Cultures of Care: Tradition and Change.' In T. Kitwood and S. Benson (eds) *The New Culture of Dementia Care*. London: Hawker.

Kitwood, T. (1997) *Dementia Reconsidered.* Buckingham: Open University Press.

Kitwood, T. and Benson, S. (eds) (1995) *The New Culture of Dementia Care.* London: Hawker.

Kitwood, T. and Bredin, K. (1992a) 'Towards a theory of dementia care: Personhood and well-being.' *Ageing and Society 12,* 3, 269–287.

Kitwood, T. and Bredin, K. (1992b) *Person to Person: A Guide to the Care of Those with Failing Mental Powers.* Loughton: Gale Centre Publications.

Kolb, D. (1983) *Experiential Learning: Experience as the Source of Learning and Development.* New Jersey: Prentice Hall.

Littlechild, R. and Blakeney, J. (1996) 'Risk and Older People.' In H. Kemshall and J. Pritchard (eds) *Good Practice in Risk Assessment and Risk Management, Volume 1.* London: Jessica Kingsley Publishers.

Martin, G.W. and Younger, D. (2001) 'Person-centred care for people with dementia: A quality audit approach.' *Journal of Psychiatric and Mental Health Nursing 8,* 443–448.

May, H., Edwards, P. and Brooker, D. (2009) *Enriched Care Planning for People with Dementia.* London: Jessica Kingsley Publishers.

Mental Capacity Act (2005) London: HMSO.

Mental Health Act (2007) London: HMSO.

Meyer, P.J. (2003) 'What Would You Do If You Knew You Couldn't Fail? Creating S.M.A.R.T. Goals.' In P.J. Meyer, *Attitude Is Everything! If You Want to Succeed Above and Beyond.* Waco, TX: Meyer Resource Group.

Murphy, C. (1994) *It Started with a Seashell.* Stirling: Dementia Services Development Centre.

National Audit Office (2010) *Improving Dementia Services in England: An Interim Report.* London: National Audit Office.

National College for School Leadership (2006) *Network Leadership in Action: Getting Started with Networked Learning Study-Visits.* Nottingham: National College for School Leadership Networked Learning Communities. Available at http://networkedlearning.ncsl.org.uk/collections/network-leadership-in-action/getting-started-with-networked-learning-study-visits-book-1.pdf, accessed on 26 March 2012.

National Institute for Health and Clinical Excellence (NICE) and the Social Care Institute for Excellence (SCIE) (2007) *Dementia: Supporting People with Dementia and Their Carers in Health and Social Care* (NICE clinical practice guideline 42: NICE/SCIE 2006). Leicester: The British Psychological Society.

Niebuhr, R. (1987) 'Serenity Prayer.' In Robert McAfee Brown (ed.) *The Essential Reinhold Niebuhr: Selected Essays and Addresses.* New Haven, CT: Yale University Press.

Nuffield Council on Bioethics (2009) *Dementia: Ethical Issues.* London: Nuffield Council on Bioethics.

Pool, J. (2007) *The Alzheimer's Society Guide to the Dementia Care Environment.* London: Alzheimer's Society.

Schön, D. (1987) *Educating the Reflective Practitioner.* San Francisco, CA: Jossey-Bass.

Sheard, D.M. (2007) *Being – An Approach to Life and Dementia.* London: Alzheimer's Society.

Sheard, D.M. (2008) *Inspiring – Leadership Matters in Dementia Care.* London: Alzheimer's Society.

Social Care Institute for Excellence (SCIE) (2009) 'What Dementia Is and What It Isn't.' In SCIE, *The Open Dementia Programme.* London: Social Care Institute for Excellence. Available at www.scie.org.uk/assets/ elearning/dementia/dementia01/resource/flash/index.html, accessed on 26 March 2012.

Sparks, D. (2004) 'From hunger aid to school reform: An interview with Jerry Sternin.' *Journal of Staff Development 25*, 1, 46–51. Available at www. positivedeviance.org/pdf/publications/From%20Hunger%20and%20 Aid%20to%20School%20Reform.pdf, accessed on 27 March 2012.

Sternin, J. (2002) 'Positive deviance: A new paradigm for addressing today's problems today.' *Journal of Corporate Citizenship 5*, 57–62.

Stokes, G. (2000) *Challenging Behaviour in Dementia: A Person-Centred Approach.* Bicester: Speechmark Publishing.

Stokes, G. (2008) *And Still the Music Plays.* London: Hawker Publications.

Walker, B. and Manterfield, S. (2010) *A Little Book of Care Planning.* Nottingham: Walker-Manterfield Associates.

Webb, G. (1995) 'Reflective practice, staff development and understanding.' *Studies in Continuing Education 17*, 1–2, 70–77.

Williams, J. and Rees, J. (1997) 'The use of "Dementia Care Mapping" as a method of evaluating care received by patients with dementia: An initiative to improve quality of life.' *Journal of Advanced Nursing 25*, 316–323.

York-Barr, J., Sommers W.A. and Ghere G.S. (2006) *Reflective Practice to Improve Schools: An Action Guide for Educators.* Thousand Oaks, CA: Corwin Press.

Index

Italic page numbers indicate figures and tables.

Aarsland, D. 59
abilities
  building on 31
  harnessing 68
  recognising 24
acceptance 28
action planning 148–150
active listening 76
Adams, T. 47
advice, giving 93
advocacy 58, 120–121
Ajzen, I. 47
Angelou, Maya 29
anger 34
anxiety 34
appraisal 78
approachability 67–68
Arin-Krupp, J. 88
Asch, S.E. 48
assessment 107–108
  of risk 139–141
assistive technology 142–143
attachment 28
attitudes, negative 44–45
autonomy 27, 33

bad practice 102–105
Ballard, C. 59
barriers
  group norms 47–50
  hopelessness 52–54
  individual habits 51–52
  learning goals 43
  limited resources 56–58
  management styles 55–56
  negative attitudes 44–46
  policies, procedures and systems 54–56
  recognising 44
  summary and conclusion 62

Beckford, M. 31
behaviour
  communicating need 134
  interpreting 132–133
  responding to problems 135–136
  triggers 133, 135–136
  see also risk
Benson, S. 48
Blakeney, J. 139
bodily needs 28
Bonaparte, Napoleon 19
Bredin, K. 31, 34
Brooker, D. 59, 108
Brooker, Dawn 20
Bryden, Christine 29, 128, 130

care leaders
  action planning 148–150
  breaking habits 51–52
  as champions 26–27
  emphasis on communication 30
  facing challenges 147–148
  information gathering 26
  minimising secondary losses of ability 22
  responsibility for well-being 34
  risk taking 56
  as role models 65–67, 100
  seeing others' perspectives 130–131
  sensitivity 46–47
  supporting learning 85–86
  validation of positive practice 50
care plans
  auditing 110
  checklist 111
  clarity of 110
  as communication tools 108–110
  structuring 110
care, quality questions 29–30
carers, support for 122–123
Chalfont, G. 31
challenges, for leaders 147–148
challenging behaviour 74–75
  understanding 128–134, 144–145

champions, care leaders as 26–27
changes
    effective strategies for 50
    information gathering 59–62
    raising awareness 58–59
    small steps 53
Chenoweth, L. 59
Christian, Debbie 26
Clarke, C.L. 138
cognitive dissonance 48
collaborative learning 67–68
comfort 28
communication
    care plan as tool 108–110
    care plans 108–112
    with external professionals 119–121
    handover meetings 114–116
    language 116–118
    of needs through behaviour 134
    non-verbal 87
    overview 107
    paying attention 26
    with relatives and friends 121–125
    and self-respect 34
    with staff 112–118
    taking and making opportunities 29–30
    underlying message 30
    verbal 112–113
    of vision 65
    written 113–114
compensating for difficulties 24
confidentiality 112
conformity, as barrier 48–49
congruence 66
consistency 66
constructive feedback 99–102
control
    of environment 27
    and well-being 33
creative brainstorming 133
creativity
    care leaders 41
    encouraging 67
    and habit 52
    service users 32
    staff 72–73
    use of resources 57
culture, development of 13, 41

damaging care practice 44
debriefing 88
dementia
    insight 74
    prevalence 13
    understanding of 20

Dementia Care Leadership Programme 14
Dementia Care Mapping (DCM) 59–60
Dementia Champions 15, 73–74
Dementia Reconsidered (Kitwood) 36
dementing illness
    course of 23
    optimal course of 23
Department of Health 20, 84
depression 34
diagnostic overshadowing 20–21
difficulties
    compensating for 24
    possible causes 21
disciplinary procedures 38, 102–105
discussions
    one-to-one 62
    problem solving 131–134

Edwards, P. 108
Eiseley, Loren C. 150
emotional needs, of staff 74–79
emotional support, for staff 75–76, 137
empathy
    with service users 129–131, 137
    with staff 128–129
empowerment, of staff 67–70
enabling 36
engagement
    with environment 30
    and well-being 31–32
Enriched Care Planning 108
environment
    engagement with 30–31
    group 31
    maintaining personhood 27
    and occupation 31
    and psychological needs 31
    and risk 142
example setting 66
exasperation, staff 75
exhaustion, staff 75
expectations 66, 97
experience, reflecting on 88
external professionals, communication with 119–121

feasibility 66
feedback
    on bad practice 102–105
    constructive 81, 99–102
    giving 101–102
    learning culture 95
    validation of positive practice 95–99
feedback mechanisms 74

feedback sandwich 101–102
feelings
    acknowledging 74–75
    empathy with service users 129–131
    empathy with staff 128–129
    problem solving in teams 131–134
    responding to 127–128
    responding to problems 135–136
    summary and conclusion 144–145
    unfixable problems 137
    working with risk *see* risk
Festinger, L. 48
Fishbein, M. 47
flexibility 41
Fossey, J. 50
freedom of movement 27, 38
friends and relatives
    communication with 121–125
    relationships with 124–125
frustration, staff 75
functioning
    actual and possible levels 22–23
    maximising potential 23–25
funding limitations 57

genuineness 28–29
Ghere, G.S. 88
goals 19
    as basis of vision 37
    dementia care 144
    holistic approach 28–31
    maintaining personhood 25–27
    maximising potential 23–25
    minimising secondary losses of ability
        20–23
    well-being 31–35
    see also objectives; vision
group environment 31
group norms 47–50
group support, for staff 78–79

habits, as barriers 51–52
handover meetings 114–116
health and safety 38
health problems, effects of 22
Heiser, Sue 116
Holden, P. 19
holistic perspective 28–31
home care, resources 57
hopelessness, as barrier 52–54
hygiene 28

identity
    and environment 27
    maintaining 25
ill-being 34
    see also well-being
importance 28
inclusion 28
individuality
    championing 26–27
    emphasising 20
    focus on 149–150
    knowledge of 45
    of staff 68–70
information gathering 25–26, 59–62,
    107–108
information, recording and using 108–110
insight, in dementia 74
insights, making use of 87–88
inspiration, of staff 37–38
interactions, personalising 27
interests, building on 31
interview questions 39
Iuppa, Nicholas 76

James, I. 50
job advertisements, wording 39
Jolley, D. 21

key points
    barriers to care 63
    communication 126
    feelings 145
    goals of care 42
    learning culture 106
    role models 82
keys 27
Kings Fund principles 37
Kitwood, Tom 13, 20, 22–23, 28, 31, 34,
    36, 44, 48
knowledge, and understanding 44–45
Kolb, D. 88, 89

labelling 117
language 46, 116–118
leadership *see* care leaders
leadership potential 72–74
leadership roles, range of 14–15
learning, collaborative 67–68
learning culture
    bad practice 102–105
    engaging staff 93–94
    feedback 95
    finding the right training 84–85

learning culture *cont.*
  giving advice 93
  observational skills 86–88
  overview 83
  reflective practice 89–94, 144
  summary and conclusion 105
  supporting learning 85–86
  validation of positive practice 95–99
  see also training
learning cycle *89*, 89–90
  blocked 90–91, *91*
Learning Walks 60–61
legislation 138
life histories 22, 25–26, 45
lighting 31
listening
  active 76
  structured 79
Littlechild, R. 139
Living Well with Dementia 20
love 28

maintaining personhood 25–27
maintaining well-being *33*
making possible 40–42
malignant social psychology 44
management styles, as barriers 55–56
Manterfield, S. 110, 112
Martin, G.W. 59
maximising potential 23–25
  partnership working *24*
May, H. 108
mealtimes 40–41
media, negative attitudes 45–46
medical issues, identifying 28
medication 121
memories, of feelings 29
Mental Capacity Act 2005 138–139
Mental Health Act 2007 138
Meyer, P.J. 149
mission statements 36
mistakes 99–100
modelling care 65–67
motivation
  questionnaire 71–72
  staff 46–47, 58, 70–72
Murphy, C. 26

National Audit Office 59
National College for School Leadership 60
National Dementia Strategy for England 20,
  84–85

National Institute for Health and Clinical
  Excellence (NICE)/SCIE 59
needs
  bodily 28
  communication through behaviour *134*
negative attitudes 44–46
Niebuhr, Reinhold 62
noise 31
non-verbal communication 87
norms, as barriers 47–50
Nuffield Council on Bioethics 139
nutrition 28

objectives
  attainability 149
  see also goals; vision
observational skills 86–88
observational tools 34–35
occupation 28, 30–31
one-to-one support 76–77
openness 43
organisational norms, as barriers 54–56
outside space, access to 31
overview, of this book 15–17

partnership working, maximising potential
  24
patience 50
pay rates 57, 58, 70
peer support 79
person centred, overuse of phrase 36–37
person-centredness
  demands on staff 28–29
  meaning of 19–20
  as relationship-based approach 28
person specifications 39
personal data, safeguarding and using 112
personal problems, staff 77
personality, influence of 22
personhood
  appreciation of 69–70
  maintaining 25–27
  of staff 36
physical disabilities, effects of 22
physical well-being 28
policies, as barriers 54–56
positive deviants 72–73
potential, maximising 23–25
practicalities, taking account of 41
practice development 59
praise 96–98
pride 32
prior experience 40

priorities
    clarity of 38
    making possible 40–42
problem solving, team-working 131–134
problems
    responding to 135–136
    unfixable 137
procedures, as barriers 54–56
professionals, negative attitudes 46
psychological needs, and environment 31
psychological well-being 28

quality of life 30–31

record keeping 113–114
recruitment, staff 39
Rees, J. 59
reflecting-in-action 94, 144
reflecting-on-action 94
reflective practice 89–94, 144
relationship-based approach 28
relationship building 26, 28
relationships
    genuine 28–29
    maintaining 28
    with relatives and friends 124–125
    and well-being 33
relatives and friends
    communication with 121–125
    relationships with 124–125
resilience, and making changes 53
resources
    as barriers 56–58
    creative use 57
respect 28
    demonstrating 66
    staff for leaders 36
    and teamwork 81
responsibilities, understanding 37–38
restrictions, avoiding unnecessary 27
rights, protection of 38, 138
risk
    assessing individual 139–141
    assistive technology 142–143
    collaborative working 143–144
    environmental adaptation 142
    harms vs.benefits 140
    management 141–142
    minimisation 27
    monitoring changes 141–142
    supporting 38
risk taking 56
role models, care leaders as 65–67, 100
routine, norms of 49

safety 27
Schön, Donald 94
seating 31
secondary losses of ability 20–23
self-expression 31–33, 34
self-respect 33, 34
sensory deficits, effects of 22
Serenity Prayer 62
service users
    empathy with 129–131, 137
    involvement in recruitment 39
    knowledge of 66–67
    spending time with 66–67
setting an example 66
shared vision 36–38
Sheard, David 28, 31
'Signs of wellbeing weekly monitoring'
    34–35, 35
silent harm 138
SMART objectives 149
Sommers, W.A. 88
space, maintaining personhood 27
staff
    acknowledging feelings 74–75
    attitudes 44–45
    communication 112–118
    disempowerment 55–56
    emotional needs 74–79
    emotional support 75–76, 137
    empathy with 128–129
    empathy with service users 129–131,
        137
    empowering 67–70
    genuineness 28–29
    group support 78–79
    harnessing strengths and abilities 68
    information gathering 26
    inspiring and guiding 36–40
    knowledge of 68, 77
    leadership potential 72–74
    morale 46–47
    motivation 46–47, 58, 70–72
    motivation questionnaire 71–72
    one-to-one support 76–77
    partnership working 68
    person specifications 39
    personal problems 77
    personal resources 69–70
    personhood 36
    power to influence 81
    prior experience 40
    rates of pay 57, 58
    recruitment 39
    role of 25

staff *cont.*
   rotation 55
   telephone contact 78
   verbal communication 112–113
staffing ratios 57
standards 97
status quo, challenging 56
Sternin, Jerry 72–73
Stokes, Graham 90–91, 133
strengths
   harnessing 68
   recognising 24
structured listening 79
supervision 78
Surr, C. 59
symptoms, understanding 44–45
systems, as barriers 54–56

taking stock 58–59
task-centred approaches 47
team building 58
team dynamics 79–81
team meetings
   group support 78–79
   staff development 73–74
team-working 34, 37–38
   problem solving 131–134
   risk management 143–144
telephone contact, with staff 78
television, constant 49
thanks 96–98
The Star Thrower (Eiseley) 150
time, making use of 30
toilets 27
training
   development of 14
   finding the right training 84–85
   induction 84
   support for new learning 85–86
   see also learning culture
trust 66, 67–68
   development of 26, 75–76
   between professionals 121
   staff for leaders 36

understanding 28, 44–45
unlearning 45–46

validation of positive practice 95–99
valuing 36
verbal communication 112–113

vision
   communicating 65
   need for 13
   shared 36–38
   underlying goals 37
   see also goals; objectives
vision statements 36
visualisation 37
   exercise 38

Walker, B. 110, 112
Warnock, Baroness M. 31
Webb, G. 100
well-being
   expressions of 31–33
   maintaining 33
   meaning of 34
   optimising 31–35
   physical 28
   psychological 28
   recognising 31–32
whistleblowing 38
whole person, addressing needs of 28–31
Williams, J. 59
written communication 113–114
'www.ebi' 100, 102, 104

'yes but…' mentality 37
York-Barr, J. 88
Younger, D. 59